ASSURANCE OF STERILITY FOR SENSITIVE COMBINATION PRODUCTS AND MATERIALS

ASSURANCE OF STERILITY FOR SENSITIVE COMBINATION PRODUCTS AND MATERIALS

New Paradigms to Bring Innovative Healthcare Products to Patients

Edited by

BYRON J. LAMBERT

STAN LAM

JOYCE M. HANSEN

TRABUE D. BRYANS

ELSEVIER

ACADEMIC PRESS

An imprint of Elsevier

Academic Press is an imprint of Elsevier
125 London Wall, London EC2Y 5AS, United Kingdom
525 B Street, Suite 1650, San Diego, CA 92101, United States
50 Hampshire Street, 5th Floor, Cambridge, MA 02139, United States
The Boulevard, Langford Lane, Kidlington, Oxford OX5 1GB, United Kingdom

Notices
Knowledge and best practice in this field are constantly changing. As new research and experience broaden our understanding, changes in research methods, professional practices, or medical treatment may become necessary.

Practitioners and researchers must always rely on their own experience and knowledge in evaluating and using any information, methods, compounds, or experiments described herein. In using such information or methods they should be mindful of their own safety and the safety of others, including parties for whom they have a professional responsibility.

To the fullest extent of the law, neither the Publisher nor the authors, contributors, or editors, assume any liability for any injury and/or damage to persons or property as a matter of products liability, negligence or otherwise, or from any use or operation of any methods, products, instructions, or ideas contained in the material herein.

Library of Congress Cataloging-in-Publication Data
A catalog record for this book is available from the Library of Congress

British Library Cataloguing-in-Publication Data
A catalogue record for this book is available from the British Library

ISBN: 978-0-12-805082-8

Publisher: Matthew Deans
Acquisition Editor: Sabrina Webber
Editorial Project Manager: John Leonard
Production Project Manager: Sojan P. Pazhayattil
Cover Designer: Mark Rogers

Typeset by SPi Global, India

Contents

Contributors

Hal Baseman
Valsource Inc., Jupiter, FL, United States

Trabue D. Bryans
BryKor, LLC, Marietta, GA, United States

Harry Frederick Bushar
Retired Statistician, Rockville, MD, United States

Joyce M. Hansen
J&J Sterility Assurance, Johnson & Johnson, Raritan, NJ, United States

Eamonn Victor Hoxey
E V Hoxey Ltd, Cirencester, United Kingdom

Stan Lam
Process and Technology Development, Stryker Neurovascular, Fremont, CA, United States

Byron J. Lambert
Assurance of Sterility Task Force, ASTF, Abbott, Temecula, CA, United States

Vu H. Le
Divisional Engineering, Abbott, Temecula, CA, United States

Andrew L. Lewis
Biocompatibles UK Ltd, a BTG International Group Company, Camberley, United Kingdom

Brad Lundahl
Johnson & Johnson Microbial Quality and Sterility Assurance, Raritan, NJ, United States

James Niederecker
R&D Quality, Abbott Vascular, Temecula, CA, United States

Michael H. Scholla
Dupont, Wilmington, DE, United States

Jane Severin
Network Partners, Warsaw, IN, United States

Marc L. Speck
R&D Quality, Abbott Vascular, Temecula, CA, United States

Donna Swenson
AAMI, Arlington, VA, United States

Steven Turtil
U.S. Food and Drug Administration/CDRH, Silver Spring, MD, United States

Jennifer Van Mullekom
Virginia Tech, Blacksburg, VA, United States

Thierry Wagner
Dupont, Luxembourg

Scott Weiss
Industrial Microbiology, Johnson & Johnson Microbiological Quality and Sterility Assurance, Raritan, NJ, United States

Foreword

The health-care industry is in a time of significant and unprecedented changes in the sterile products. New therapies are being developed that combine the benefit of drug products with the specificity of delivery devices. Global health authorities are becoming more influential in the preparation of guidance setting expectations for improved process and contamination control. Innovative manufacturing, sterilization and data acquisition technologies are available, and the promises of new technologies and modalities are being constantly introduced. Continuous manufacturing, automation, and manufacturing intelligence are lowering our reliance on and concern for the variability of human performance. Simpler standardized clean room spaces equipped with rapid process monitoring, testing, and manufacturing intelligence data gathering enables improved manufacturing reliability. Throughout this journey, there is a growing recognition that traditional product testing, process monitoring, and validation may not be the most effective means to ensure sterile product quality.

Additional business factors are shaping the industry concurrently with the advances in technology. Drug and health-care product shortages are shifting public health policies to emphasize product availability, affordability, and sustainability. Industry understands that quality processes resulting in higher yields, increased productivity, and reduced failures makes good business sense. The improved profits in turn encourages increased investment in innovative technologies and the adoption of novel manufacturing strategies and methodologies.

The opportunities that result from these significant changes increase the use of technology for manufacturing as well as scientifically based process control. This provides a vehicle for new approaches for innovative process improvements incorporating the scientific risk-based approaches encouraged by regulators to justify the design and manufacture products approval.

Improvement which challenges the status quo often originates from asking those critical "why and why not" questions. It is essential that those responsible for planning, designing, and manufacturing health-care products employ critical thinking for the efficient development of effective products.

Combination therapies and products emerge to provide effective and affordable health-care options to our patients. A large proportion of these products are required to be either sterile or low bioburden. New products and therapies will require new approaches to product development and process control. This is happening in a time of expanded global distribution and manufacturing, requiring a more diversified level of regulatory awareness, understanding, and compliance strategies.

There are challenges ahead for those developing and manufacturing sterile combination products. Are we prepared for such innovation and change? Is our industry, including those who regulate it, equipped to develop, manufacture, test, distribute and control the quality of these new products efficiently and effectively to best serve our patients?

This book has been written to help the reader recognize, understand, and meet these challenges, from the development, manufacture, test, and control the constantly improving innovative combination products. It presents the background and the requirements for the rapidly emerging field of sensitive combination products through an overview of the history, definition, and classification strategies used by regulatory bodies, and an exploration of traditional and novel sterilization methods instrumental for successful combination products.

To better understand where we must go, we must start by defining our destination: the sterility and sterility assurance of sensitive combination products. The use of sterility assurance terms across the health-care sectors, including sterility assurance level and probability of a non-sterile unit must be fully understood to understand the true risk to the patient. To that end, chapters of the book explore the current and emerging disciplines use to produce products to achieve and maintain sterility assurance. This includes sterilization, aseptic processing, packaging, and a thorough discussion and exploration of the development, validation and routine control of contamination, and process control of health-care products.

The role of bioburden control and process validation throughout the design and defense of the contamination control strategy are explained. It starts with the identification of product quality attributes and related requirements, then leads to the development of process steps to attain, validate, maintain, and monitor those product quality attributes, through the critical process parameter including the sterilization of product and the prevention of contamination.

Chapters of the book provide the history of radiation sterilization, ethylene oxide sterilization, and heat sterilization, an overview of the principles and methods for validating the logarithmic reduction in microbial load by a terminal sterilization process, traditional overkill approach, and bioburden-based methods that are increasing in importance due to environmental as well as product compatibility reasons.

The chapter on aseptic processing lays out a prudent strategy focused on aseptic processing and sterility by design. It introduces the powerful line-of-sight process control approach which leads to robust user requirements. Practical aseptic practices and environmental monitoring cleanroom design approaches are discussed, including aseptic barrier systems, e.g., isolators, and critical utilities. Practical process simulation design guidance is recommended using case studies to illustrate the principles.The chapter ends with a discussion of quality risk management and risk-based critical thinking and an overview of new technologies and perspectives in the field of aseptic processing.

The essential aspects of sterile combination product packaging and container closure design are explored in chapters as an essential means to the maintenance of sterility throughout the storage, handling and use. Microbial barriers, packaging sterilization compatibility, labeling, and storage/transport requirements for materials and package components are provided. Design and development requirements are delineated, along with those for aseptic presentation. Packaging system performance and stability requirements are then discussed along with validation requirements.

A key chapter focuses on the fundamental concepts of hospital-acquired infection (HAI) and the related issues surrounding the handling and use of health-care products. This topic is critical in the discussion of the overall sterility risk to the patient and alternate ways to determine sterility assurance levels. An analysis of the breakdown and rates of HAIs enables an understanding of the relative magnitude of these issues. By discussing the root causes of HAIs-principally related to clinical personnel and practices, and surveying case studies, prevention strategies can be determined and recommended.

As members of the global health-care product community, our primary objective is ensuring the health and welfare of patients. It is through the understanding of patient needs that new products are developed. It is through identification of the required quality attributes of those products that processes are designed. It is through recognition of the variables of those processes that control strategies are employed. It is through the utilization of innovative technologies that products are improved.

In this way, awareness of patient needs, product requirements, processes variables, and available technology result in addressing today's and tomorrow's health-care challenges more effectively. Books such as *Assurance of Sterility for Sensitive Combination Products and Materials* provide a path for reaching that level of awareness and thus help our industry achieve our goal of improving patient welfare through improved health-care products.

Hal Baseman
Valsource, Jupiter, FL, United States

CHAPTER 1

Introduction: Sterilization or aseptic processing of single use combination products

Joyce M. Hansen[a], Trabue D. Bryans[b]
[a]J&J Sterility Assurance, Johnson & Johnson, Raritan, NJ, United States
[b]BryKor, LLC, Marietta, GA, United States

Contents

1.1 Introduction

New patient treatment options continue to drive the need for the development of combination products. Sterility assurance innovation is critical to bring these combination products to market. This innovation requires sterility assurance professionals to collaborate across the broad spectrum of the demands of the healthcare industry. Not only does a successful sterility assurance professional need to be an expert in their field, but also they need to be aware of the broad challenges and opportunities associated with bringing a combination product to the market. This book provides an overview as well as introduces exciting new opportunities in each industry sector. The sectors addressed include combination products and their design, terminal sterilization, aseptic processing, packaging, healthcare practices as well as the worldwide regulatory environment. The topics associated with each sector are introduced with the perspective of facilitating the development of innovative new combination products.

Combination products emerged in the 1990s to reduce the potential for infection and the time healthcare providers needed to treat patients. Original combination products typically consisted of a means of connecting multiple products to reduce the manipulations required. Over the last few decades, combination products have evolved to consist of a combination of medical devices, biologics, pharmaceuticals, and electronics to support the next level of patient care.

Assurance of Sterility for Sensitive Combination Products and Materials
https://doi.org/10.1016/B978-0-12-805082-8.00001-3

The regulatory evolution of combination products has provided manufacturers with an opportunity to envision a new subset of products that utilize various combinations of medical devices, biologics, pharmaceuticals, active electronics, and/or bioresorbables in unique manners. Therefore, the regulatory climate for combination products necessitated the use of a blend of requirements that would be specific for the appropriate combination of medical device, biologics, and/or pharmaceutical products.

Until recently, healthcare products were typically classified as medical devices, biologics, or pharmaceuticals. The different classifications of products were traditionally regulated through different parts of regulatory agencies, which have for years operated independently. The requirements for different categories of products did not typically involve coordination across agencies. The development of combination products has required that manufacturers as well as regulators learn to navigate the diverse requirements across the different agencies.

A successful sterility assurance professional—with the convergences of this changing regulatory landscape—requires the ability to connect the dots across the different sectors of the industry that have traditionally, all too often, been in silos. Combination products may need terminal sterilization and/or aseptic processing; and sterilization professionals need to understand both. The majority of healthcare risks to patients include those associated with healthcare facilities themselves; hence, sterilization professionals need to understand how the product is used in the healthcare facilities and the magnitude of hospital-acquired infections (HAI).

One of the unique value streams of this book is its perspective integrating discussion of sterility assurance topics across industry sectors. This presents a terminology challenge since different sectors use different but related terminology. This is addressed as follows.

1.2 Sterility assurance terminology

The term 'sterile' is generally defined as an absolute state, for example, *the absence of viable microorganisms.* Different terms are used in different sterility assurance sectors as follows:

Sterility assurance level (SAL) is specific to terminal sterilization, defined as the "probability of a single viable microorganism occurring on an item after sterilization."

Probability of a non-sterile unit (PNSU) is sometimes used for terminally sterilized components feeding into an aseptic process.

Contamination rate is used to describe the results of process simulations in aseptic processing validations.

The definition of SAL is the probability of survival of a single microorganism. Microbiological reduction associated with terminal sterilization processes is expressed by an exponential function. The values of SAL and PNSU are a negative power to the base 10. All of the terminal sterilization methods explicitly use the term SAL and this mathematical construct in the validation scheme. This construct differs from the term PNSU, which is based on a product being non-sterile, whether due to a single microorganism or multiple microorganisms.

Typically, the first step in the development of a new product is understanding patient needs. Based on this information, an initial product design is developed, and integral to the product design is the determination of whether the product can withstand a terminal sterilization process. This is particularly challenging for combination products because of the need to use different materials that might not be suitable for traditional overkill sterilization processes. Materials such as active electronics, bioresorbable materials, and biologics are particularly challenging. The option of aseptic processing can be considered after demonstrating that the product cannot be terminally sterilized. The regulatory agencies and industries are adapted to accommodate sterilization challenges of combination products that cannot be terminally sterilized by developing aseptic processing standards for solid combination products (e.g., ISO 13408-7). Chapters in this book explore the options for both terminal sterilization and aseptic processing, as well as the selection of an alternate SAL for those products that cannot be terminally sterilized to an SAL of 10^{-6}.

The underpinning behind the development of sterilization modalities, aseptic processing, packaging, and healthcare acquired infection is the concept of infection risk to the patient. The independent evolution of the sectors resulted in different methods and vocabulary to quantify the risk. A fundamental statistical approach is presented to attempt to bridge these assessments. The goal of the Risk to Patient chapter is to open the dialog between groups so that informed scientific-based decisions can be made.

Regardless of the method of providing a sterile product—terminal sterilization or aseptic processing—the primary packaging is required to maintain the integrity of the sterile claim. Primary packaging is intended to provide the sterile barrier throughout the product shelf life, including handling and distribution activities. Packaging for a combination product might include both traditional trays and pouches for medical devices, as well as traditional containers/closures used for biologics or pharmaceuticals.

One of the major challenges for combination products is how to achieve the sterile label claim. This challenge dictates the choice of the process used to assure sterility, and the level of manufacturing controls needed for production. This challenge also has resulted in the opportunity to not only reevaluate the traditional SAL but also consider the applicability and risk of alternate SALs. Navigating this challenge has required that manufacturers as well as regulators collaborate on how to achieve the sterile label claim.

Combination products and the associated regulatory aspects are dynamic topics that continue to evolve driven by the new types of products that will be needed for the future. This book will help equip sterility assurance professionals to address new opportunities in order to ensure that patients receive the optimal products with optimal risk-based sterilization solutions.

CHAPTER 2

Sensitive combination products: Devices, pharmaceuticals, and biologics

Andrew L. Lewis
Biocompatibles UK Ltd, a BTG International Group Company, Camberley, United Kingdom

Contents

2.1 Introduction to combination products

Combination products have been in existence for many decades now but since the turn of the millennia, there has been a more rapid evolution of complex therapeutic products that fall between the lines of the classic definitions of a drug, device, or biological product. This prompted the FDA (Food and Drug Administration) to form the Office of Combination Products in 2002 in an effort to act as a resource and provide guidance to industry, to classify, assign, and oversee the regulation of products that fall within their definition of a combination product (see Fig. 2.1).

Manufacturers can formally request designation for their products based on arguments that define its principal function within the body, which determines which branch within FDA will take lead on regulation of the product. The FDA follows a clear algorithm that first considers the greatest contribution to the overall intended therapeutic effect of the combination products—the so-called primary mode of action (PMOA). Sometimes this in itself can be unclear, in which case they turn to the agency that either

Assurance of Sterility for Sensitive Combination Products and Materials
https://doi.org/10.1016/B978-0-12-805082-8.00002-5

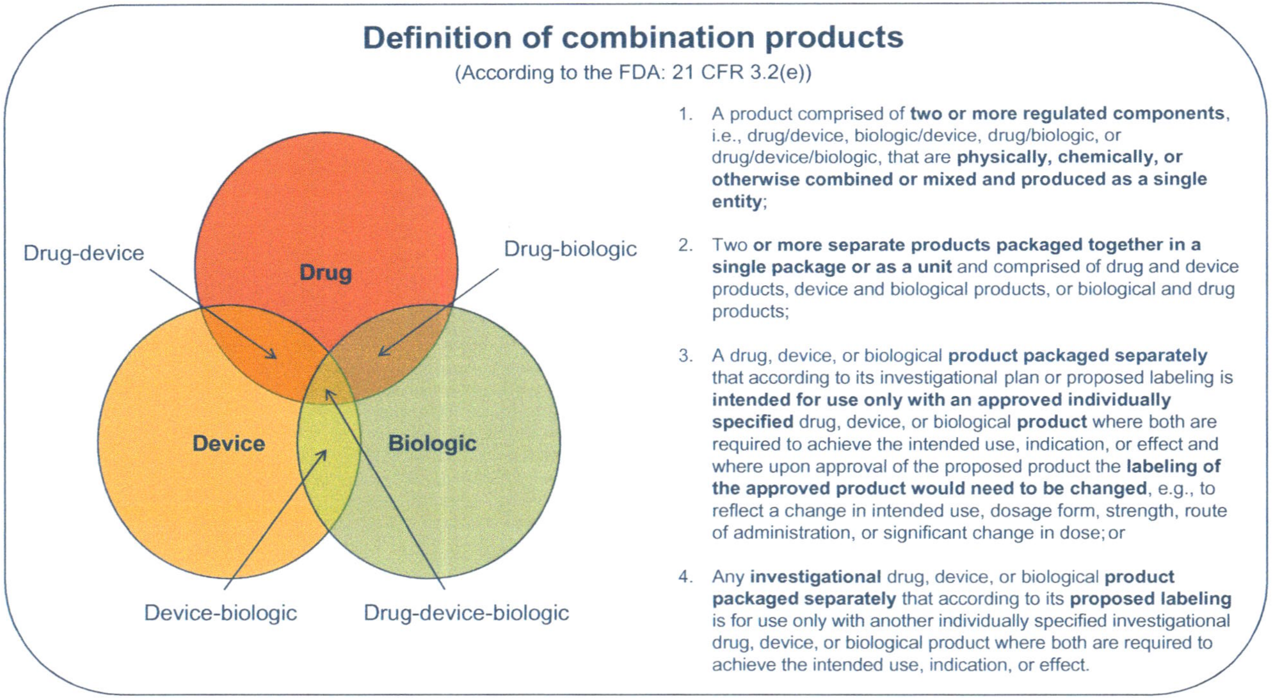

Fig. 2.1 Definition of combination products.

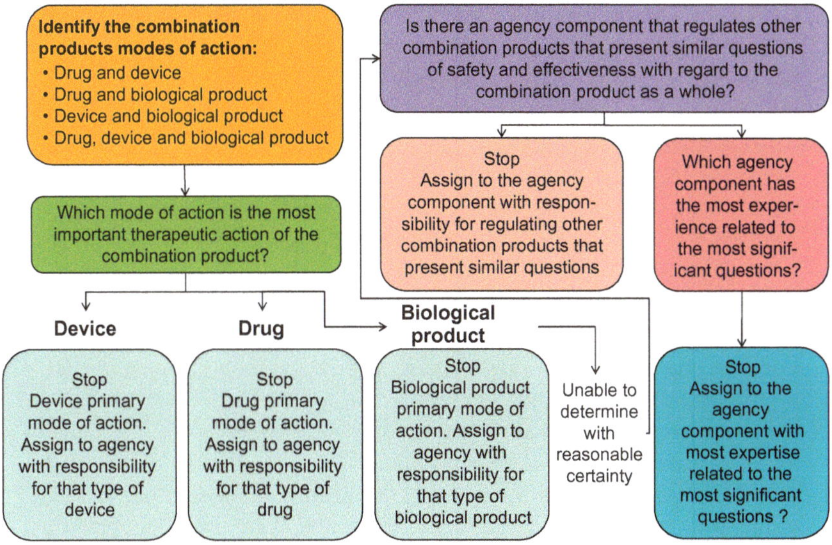

Fig. 2.2 Primary mode of action assignment algorithm.

deals with similar safety and efficacy questions as the product under consideration, or has expertise in the most significant safety and efficacy questions for the product (see Fig. 2.2).

Case study 1: PMOA determination for drug-eluting beads

An interesting case study to consider PMOA determination is that of drug-eluting beads (DEBs) developed for the treatment of tumors [1, 2]. Microspheres have been used for many years to treat both benign and malignant tumors, by injecting them through microcatheters directly into the arterial blood supply that feeds the growth. They subsequently flow into the vessels until they lodge, causing a blockage of the vessel and starving the tumor of its blood supply and hence oxygen and nutrients. These embolization microspheres are therefore classified as medical devices as they physically occlude blood vessels. In the past decade there has been an evolution in clinical practice to the use of microspheres that can be loaded with chemotherapeutic agents in the hospital pharmacy prior to a procedure [3], such that when the microspheres are injected they flow and occlude the vessels as before but subsequently elute and deliver chemotherapeutic agent over a sustained period of time. As at the point of use this product is a combination of a device and a drug, it fulfils the definition of a combination product. As embolization is the PMOA followed by a secondary drug action, the product falls within the primary jurisdiction of the FDAs

Continued

Center for Devices and Radiologic Health (CDRH). This is analogous to the case for drug-eluting stents (DES), where the PMOA is maintenance of the arterial lumen and secondarily, delivery of a drug to prevent restenosis in the vessel. The DEBs, however, have also been evaluated in the treatment of other solid tumors; recent preclinical [4, 5] and clinical studies have evaluated the direct injection of DEBs into the resection cavity left post surgical removal of a brain tumor. In this case, there is no physical arterial occlusion involved; the microsphere acts to hold and deliver the drug locally into the tissue in which it is injected, the primary therapeutic effect being provided by the action of the chemotherapeutic. In this case, therefore, despite the product being identical to that used to treat liver metastases by embolization, the route of administration and hence the primary therapeutic effect is different, and the combination product has a drug PMOA and would be regulated as medicinal product [hence, in the United States by the Center for Drug Evaluation and Research (CDER)].

As demonstrated in this case study, the term combination product describes the entity used to treat a patient at the point of use and can therefore be essentially considered as including:

- chemically or physically combined products (e.g., DES, transdermal patches, metered dose inhalers, and prefilled syringes);
- co-packaged products (e.g., drug or biological product packaged with a delivery device, surgical kits, and first-aid kits);
- "cross-labeled" products [e.g., photosensitizing drug and activating laser source, iontophoretic drug delivery patch, and controller (both labeled specifically for use with one another)]

If the two components of the combination product are manufactured separately and co-packaged or cross-labeled, each component can be developed independent of the other by the conventional methods used for their manufacture. Where the components are physically or chemically combined into one product and packaged together, a strategy must be employed to ensure that the combined end product can be satisfactorily sterilized by a method that will ensure that none of the components are degraded or altered by the sterilization step. The remainder of this chapter will focus on considerations for the sterilization of this type of sensitive combination product.

2.2 Considerations for sterilization of combination products

Primum non nocere—"first do no harm" is the fundamental code adopted by a physician when considering patient treatment options; and which is similarly inherent to all medicines and devices provided to physicians by their manufacturers. One generic risk associated with all products entering the hospital environment, particularly if intended to be used in an invasive

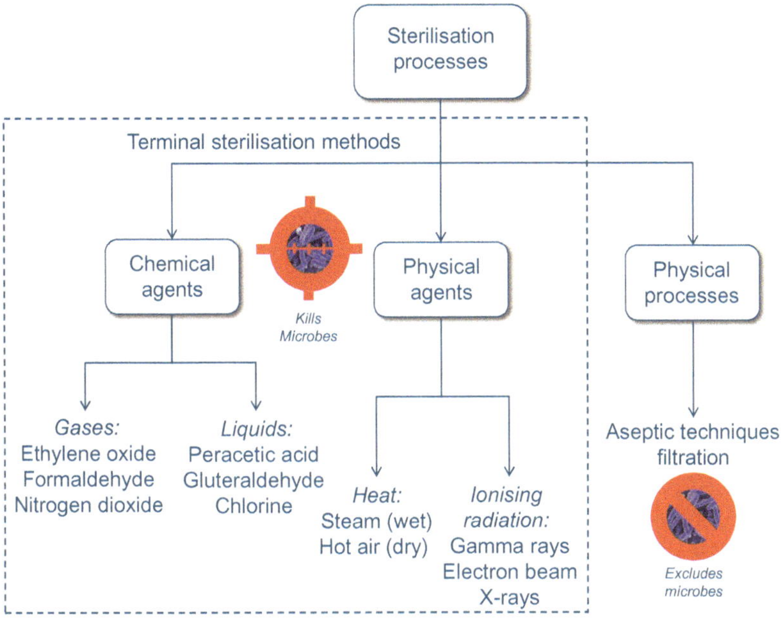

Fig. 2.3 Methods of sterilization.

treatment or for implantation within the body, is that of product-related infections [6, 7]. The manufacturers usually safeguard against this risk by sterilizing their products using one of a selection of commonly used processes to eliminate bioburden (Fig. 2.3). The most manufacturing-efficient route is to validate a terminal sterilization process in which the product within its final sterile packaging is subjected to a step designed to kill the vast majority of microbial contaminants associated with the product [8]. The extent of the reduction in microbial count is somewhat related to the function of the product: if it is not required to contact open wounds or other surfaces that could provide a conduit to infection on or in the body, then it is accepted that the probability of contamination should be less than one in a thousand products (a sterility assurance level, or SAL of 10^{-3}). Otherwise, if risk of infection is even remotely possible, the SAL increases to one in a million (SAL of 10^{-6}), which is the requirement for most combination products given the nature of these products and their intended use.

Terminal sterilization can involve the use of gamma radiation, electron beam, heat (steam) or biologically reactive chemical vapors such as ethylene oxide. All of these processes are designed to destroy complex biological structures with efficiency and hence, as products become more complex in their composition, they too can become affected by the sterilization process.

Gamma and electron beam sterilization work on the same basic principle that high energy radiation damages and breaks DNA of living organisms, such as bacteria, resulting in cell death. Naturally, therefore, this mode of sterilization may not be a good choice for treatment of a combination product that is designed to deliver complex biomacromolecules such as oligonucleotides, RNAs, or DNAs. A further drawback of terminal sterilization is that remnants of the dead microbes remain associated with the product post-processing. The cell wall of Gram-negative bacteria is composed of lipopolysaccharides that are released upon death and these so-called endotoxins can elicit a significant immune reaction. Hence, demonstration of endotoxin levels within recommended specification limits are also generally required for products sterilized in this manner. Terminal sterilization is discussed in more details later in Chapter 3. A less attractive alternative to terminal sterilization is the use of aseptic techniques, which are inherently more labor-intensive and hence expensive and do not share the benefits of robust process control and a high degree of sterility assurance recognized with terminal sterilization. This, however, might be the only option for a complex advanced medicinal product with cellular components for instance and is the reason why there have been some advances in the guidance provided to the sterilization standards community in this area. The topic of aseptic processing is covered in great detail later in Chapter 4.

2.2.1 Drug-enhanced devices

Drug-enhanced devices are a class of combination product in which the functionality, efficacy, or performance of the device is enhanced by the presence of a therapeutic agent. The drug can be added to address a particular issue that is associated with the use of the device, or to augment the use of the device, including examples such as

- an antiproliferative agent to prevent tissue regrowth (in-stent restenosis) induced by the placement of a stent in the artery;
- an anti-infective agent delivered from an orthopedic cement to prevent infection following surgical implantation of a prosthesis;
- an anti-inflammatory to reduce the inflammation and fibrotic reaction around a hernia-repair mesh that might affect its flexibility when implanted;
- an anti-inflammatory to reduce the inflammation and fibrosis around pacemaker electrodes to make their removal less traumatic;
- a chemotherapeutic delivered from an embolization device to kill those cells that do not die as a consequence of the nutrient and oxygen reduction

The simplest form of this type of combination product would take an existing, approved drug and device and combine them. Ideally in this scenario, the drug should also be approved for the indication in which is it being used, by the same route of administration and with the same mechanism of action. There are normally, however, a range of new questions that arise as a consequence of using a device to mediate local delivery of a therapeutic that must be addressed in order to demonstrate continued safety and efficacy of the combined product.

Case study 2: Sterilization of DES

The drug may be distributed throughout the device itself (as for the DEB or an antibiotic-containing cement) or be contained in matrix such as a biomedical polymer coating, usually at the interface where the device would contact the body. The DES commonly employ this approach which allows for a consistent dose of drug to be applied along the length of the stent and concentrated on the outer surface where the device expands into contact with the vessel wall. There are a wide variety of biomedical polymers in use in these types of applications, some of which are biostable and inert, others are designed to bioresorb within the body over defined time period. In the case of biodegradable polymers, the matrices themselves may be sensitive to the processes of sterilization and premature degradation could be initiated if the wrong process is selected (see Fig. 2.4) [9, 10].

Clearly from Fig. 2.4, the hot, humid EtO vapor environment is not a good choice for polymers that degrade by hydrolytic mechanisms. As an alternative, the effects of electron beam sterilization of similar paclitaxel poly(DL-lactide-*co*-glycolide) (PLG) matrices of COSTAR stents

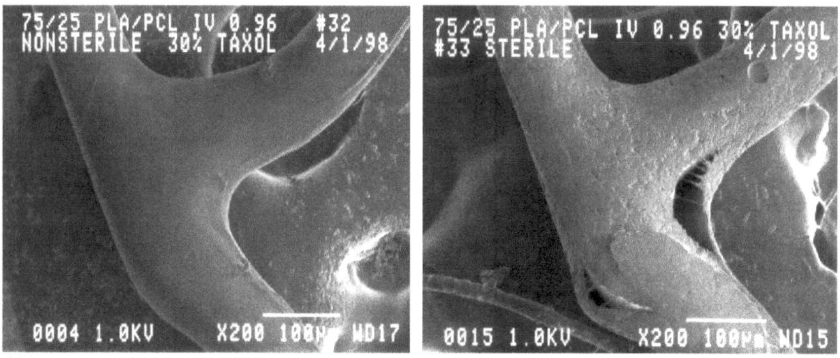

(A) (B)

Fig. 2.4 Scanning Electron Micrographs of Paclitaxel loaded Poly(lactic acid)/(caprolactone) coated coronary stent (A) before and (B) after ethylene oxide sterilization [9]. Note the heavily pitted surface and delamination of the coating from the strut surface post-sterilization.

have been investigated and numerous drug degradation products have been detected in a β-radiation dose-dependent manner, together with polymer degradants [11]. Combined LC-MS-MS analysis of these DES post-sterilization indicated that water addition and oxidative processes together with the isomerization were largely responsible for the degradation of the drug; so tight control of the combined product specification may be necessary to prevent catalytic amounts of water adversely affecting downstream processes. In general, however, many small molecules coated onto DES have been shown to be stable to gamma irradiation which remains a mainstay sterilization process. Although larger biological entities tend to be more sensitive to all modes of sterilization, it was reported that stents coated with polymer containing the antibody fragment GPIIb/IIa inhibitor, abiciximab (or c7e3) absorbed within it, maintained its antiplatelet effect even after sterilization and storage for several months [12]. The selection of a suitable method is therefore trial and error and very much depends on the individual components selected.

Case study 3: Sterilization of drug-eluting embolization beads

In the case of the DEBs described earlier, the embolization device on its own presented hydrated in buffer in glass vials and is terminally sterilized using steam. Testing was necessary to demonstrate that the steam did not induce any degradation of the material and that the device dimensions were unchanged and remained the same as per the specification and product labeling. The steam sterilization process was validated using inoculation standards to prove that all samples within the sterilizer chamber experienced sufficient heat to guarantee a 10^{-6} SAL. Endotoxin levels were also measured and specifications set to ensure that the amount of bioburden introduced during manufacture was at acceptably low level.

A preloaded version of the DEB was developed in which the drug was loaded into the microspheres during manufacturing and provided to physicians as the combined product. When this product format was initially prototyped in a hydrated form in vials and steam sterilized as per the device alone, the drug underwent complete degradation. A lyophilization processes had to be developed to remove all moisture from the microspheres after the drug was loaded, and the combination sterilized as a dry free-flowing powder in vials by gamma irradiation. For this process, it was necessary to demonstrate that the additional special processes employed did not affect either device or drug component and that when the combination was re-hydrated in water at the point of use, the product attributes were the same as that supplied separately and combined in the pharmacy. Not only did this involve validating a new sterilization method, but also shelf-life testing had to be repeated as the product format and primary packaging had both changed. This product has not yet been commercialized, however, a first-in-man clinical evaluation of a DEB preloaded with the multi-tyrosine kinase inhibitor vandetanib [13] has been approved by the Medicines and Healthcare Products Regulatory Agency (MHRA) in early 2017.

2.2.2 Drug delivery systems: Traditional and novel

Combination products that are classified as drug delivery systems are those in which the PMOA is that of the drug and the device is designed to improve the convenience and comfort of administration and improving efficacy by targeting or localizing delivery. Traditional systems include drugs combined or packaged together with injection devices to improve convenience, such as prefilled syringes, pen-based systems, and drug pumps. The novel drug delivery systems would normally enable drug to be delivered via a nonclassical route of delivery [other than oral or parenteral (subcutaneous or intravenous)]. Examples of this specific class of combination product are as follows:

- transdermal or intradermal injection systems;
- transdermal patches;
- metered dose inhalers;
- implantable drug-eluting polymer disks for tumor treatments;
- implantable drug-eluting polymer rods releasing contraceptives;
- varicose vein sclerosing foam generating device

Where the drug and the delivery system are packaged separately, sterilization is possible using the traditional approaches used for the individual components. If the drug and delivery system are combined as one during manufacturing and sold as a unit, then that combined product will need to be sterilized by a method suitable to ensure the appropriate SAL and without adverse effects on either component that would alter their safety profile or performance. Indeed, the finished product may be sterilized by multiple different sterilization processes throughout its manufacturing cycle in order to provide sterility to each of the separate components. For example, a drug-delivery device consisting of a vial of drug, water for injection (WFI), and a syringe requires that the device component is sterilized without contamination of the drug or water. One approach to achieving this could be to obtain the syringe components presterilized by gamma irradiation and the WFI may then be sterilized by steam once contained in the closed barrel of the syringe. The drug vial will be sterilized by filtration during manufacture and then combined with the syringe in a kit which will need all external surfaces sterilized in its final format. It is possible to modify existing processes to achieve this without adversely affecting the contents of the syringe and vial. Mild EtO processing cycles employing shallow vacuums, low temperatures, low gas (H_2O_2 or NO_2) concentrations, or reduced exposure times have been developed for this type of purpose, which maintain sterility and provide a route to manufacture of such drug-device combination that otherwise could be problematic.

Case study 4: Sterilization of Varithena (polidocanol injectable microfoam) 1%

Varithena (polidocanol injectable microfoam) 1% is a drug-device combination product in which a canister device fitted with a filter stack generates a microfoam with a defined bubble size distribution of polidocanol solution and an oxygen:carbon dioxide gas mixture [14]. This unique product has an excellent balance of foam stability to allow handling, administration, and injection into a varicose vein, with enough cohesive property to displace the blood from the vessel while collapsing the vein due to the sclerosing action of the polidocanol surfactant. The low nitrogen gas mixture quickly disperses in the body to reduce any adverse effects of bubbles circulating around the body and in particular transient ischemic attacks from bubbles that transit to the brain. The PMOA is that of the drug action on the vessel wall, the device is responsible for reproducible creation of the stable microfoam to a defined specification.

The sterilization of this drug-device combination product is a classic example of how long development programs that can span over a decade will have changes in personnel, suppliers, product requirements and specifications will lead to a manufacturing process that would be quite different from a program that did not have these changes. Development programmes that extend over long periods are at risk of the ever-changing regulatory environment which can result in having to repeat certain performance tests to revised standards, as well as new technologies that obtain approval in the intervening time changing the requirements and raising the bar for data.

Fig. 2.5 shows an outline flowchart for the basic steps involved in the manufacture of the Varithena (polidocanol injectable microfoam) 1% combination product. What is evident from this chart is that despite the product undergoing terminal steam sterilization, there are a number of other intermediate sterilization steps involved. The valve assemblies that are used in the canisters are created in a controlled environment but they are gamma irradiated to reduce bioburden prior to them entering a clean room environment. Exploratory work indicated that there was a risk that the polidocanol may undergo some degradation if sterilized in the presence of oxygen and so the product was split between two canisters, one containing the oxygen

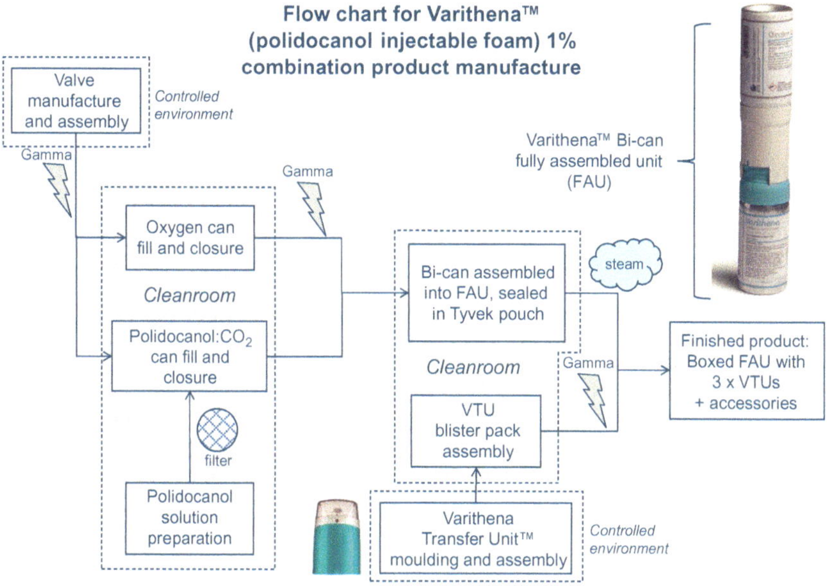

Fig. 2.5 Flow chart for the manufacture of Varithena (polidocanol injectable foam) 1% drug-device combination product manufacture.

gas and the other polidocanol solution and CO_2, to be sterilized as a bi-can assembly and the gases combined at the point of use. A decision was originally taken to continue to gamma sterilize the oxygen canister once filled and sealed but not the polidocanol canister. This was written into the procedures and shelf-life data generated; this provides somewhat of a barrier moving forwards in the process development, and if that superfluous gamma irradiation step is to be removed, a great deal of work is required to justify this to regulatory bodies and to generate new shelf-life data. The final assembled product is co-packaged with the Varithena Transfer Units needed to administer the foam from the activated canister (which itself undergoes a separate gamma sterilization) and the whole product is terminally steam sterilized. Decisions taken early on and changes to the design process have led to an over-cumbersome process that is extremely difficult to change. Moreover, extensive work has had to be undertaken to demonstrate that the components of the finished unit are not adversely affected by the several sterilization steps they are subjected to through the manufacturing process. Ideally, learn as much about the product requirements through the target product profile up front, spend time planning and designing a lean and efficient process, execute in a timely fashion, and minimize change as much as possible on the way.

2.2.3 Regenerative medical devices with biologics

Biologics (sometimes also referred to as biological drugs or agents) may be diagnostic, preventive, or therapeutic in nature. These products are generally developed and manufactured through biological processes using, for instance, bacterial, animal, or human sources, and include entities of varying degrees of complexity from sugars, proteins and nucleic acids, through to cells, blood, and other tissues. The major classes of these products include vaccines grown in cell culture, products obtained through viral gene therapy, those extracted from living systems or produced by recombinant DNA methods. Drug-biologic combination products include regenerative medicinal products that combine devices with biologically active substances to facilitate healing and regenerate damaged tissues. The device often serves as a scaffolding for the growth of the biologic component and the product is often an implant; this type of product may also be classified for use in tissue engineering. Examples of device-biologic combinations as follows:

- human fibroblast-derived dermal substitute (e.g., dermagraft);
- spinal fusion cages with recombinant human bone morphogenetic proteins;

Case study 5: Novel method for protein stabilization

A German biotech company, Leukocare AG, has developed technologies that enable the stabilization of proteins during production, sterilization by irradiation, and subsequently during storage. The technologies are known as stabilizing and protecting solutions (SPS), which can be applied to medical devices, biopharmaceuticals, vaccines, and diagnostic products (Fig. 2.6) [15]. SPS technology is a combination of 5–8 different excipients that form a thin protective amorphous coating around proteins during the drying process, increasing stability during storage and protecting the sensitive protein conformation during gamma, *E*-beam or EtO sterilization processes. The protective SPS layer is washed away when it comes in contact with water or body fluids prior to the application of the product, the original functionality of the proteins being restored. Proof of concept has been demonstrated with small peptide, oligonucleotides, enzymes, growth factors, and even antibodies such as IgM. This technology could therefore be of particular interest in the development of sensitive combination products in which a biologic is combined with a device and may offer a route to terminal sterilization that would not normally be possible due to deactivation of the biologic.

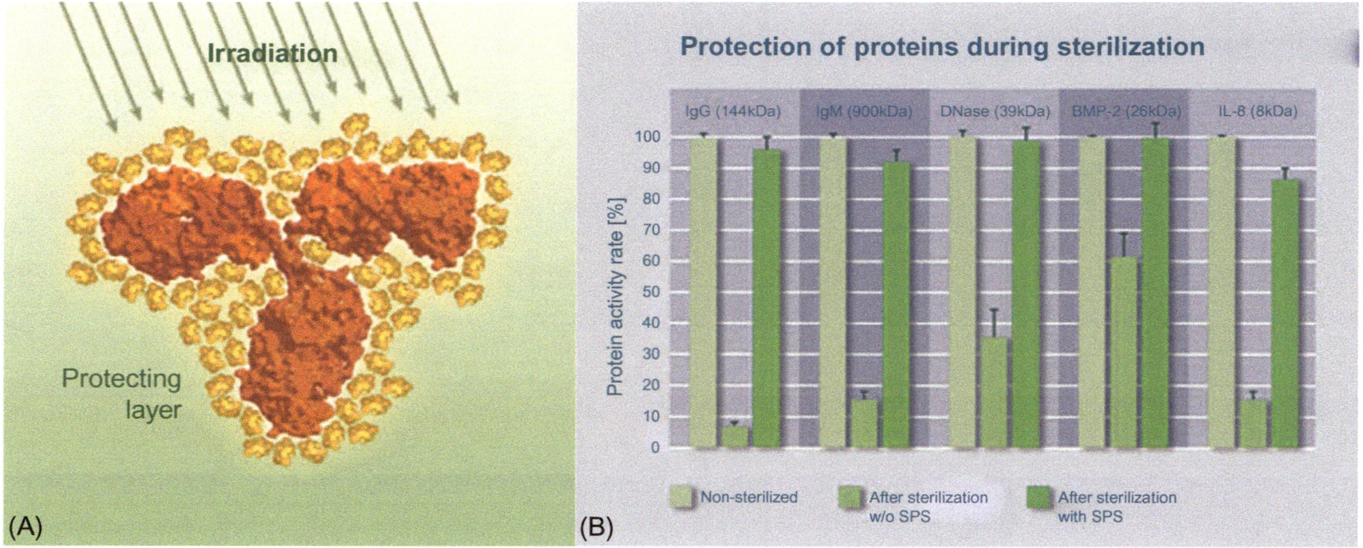

Fig. 2.6 (A) SPS stabilize the 3-D conformation of proteins, excluding water and protecting from chemical and physical stress during sterilization. (B) SPS have been shown to protect a range of functional biomolecules from 8 to 900 kDA, exposed to 25 kGy irradiation.

- autologous chondrocytes and scaffold for the repair of cartilage defects;
- autologous cell therapy and delivery device to treat cardiovascular disease;
- cultured bone marrow cells and bone void filler with handling agent for bone repair;
- artificial replacement organs (e.g., bioartificial pancreas).

The very nature of biologics makes them difficult to provide in a sterile form, in particular those containing live cellular components. Protein-based therapeutics need to maintain their sensitive three-dimensional conformations in order to remain physiologically active, which can be a significant challenge during production and sterilization processes and can also adversely affect the product shelf life. Physical and chemical degradation, destabilization, and aggregation of proteins can all occur as a consequence of changes in temperature, exposure to radiation, and initiation of hydrolytic processes during manufacture.

Case study 6: Sterilization of a spinal fusion system

The Medtronic Infuse Bone Graft/LT-CAGE lumbar tapered fusion device is a device-biologic combination product for certain spinal fusion procedures in patients with degenerative disc disease. The product is composed of a bone graft kit containing an absorbable collagen scaffold (ACS), a lyophilized bone morphogenetic protein (rhBMP-2) plus accessories, which is labeled for use with the LT-CAGE threaded implant-grade titanium alloy (Ti-6Al-4V) device (Fig. 2.7). At the point of use, the rhBMP-2 is reconstituted in sterile water and soaked into the ACS matrix; this is then rolled and inserted into the hollow interior section of the threaded titanium implant to form the complete combination product (titanium fixation device—collagen scaffold device—protein biologic, Fig. 2.7D). Two of these assemblies are then inserted and screwed into place between the two vertebrae where the disc has been damaged. The protein elutes from the ACS in a controlled and sustained manner over time, encouraging the in-growth of bone through the windows in the fixation device and eventually filling the space as the ACS resorbs, creating a bone bridge between the vertebrae [16].

Sterilization of this product is a little simplified in that the three main components of this combination product are all sterilized separately by different methods and provided in a kit or labeled for use together. The titanium fixation cage is sold separately and can be terminally sterilized by any of the conventional sterilization methods that will not affect the alloy, such as gamma irradiation. The ACS manufacture involves lyophilization of a dispersion of bovine Achilles tendon collagen followed by cross-linking

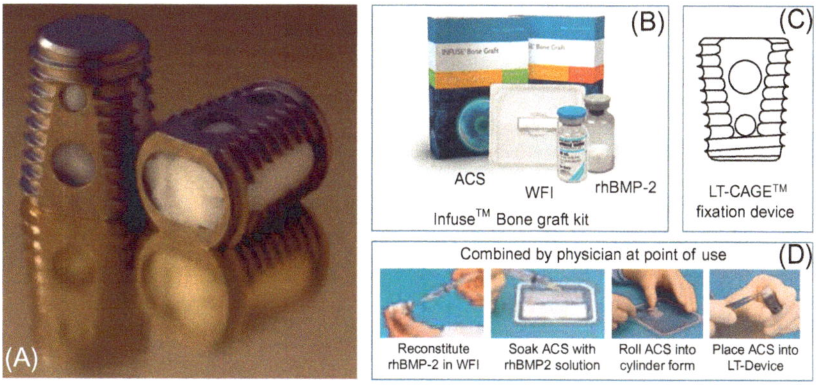

Fig. 2.7 (A) The Medtronic Infuse™ Bone Graft/LT-CAGE™ Lumbar Tapered Fusion Device in its combined form; (B) the Infuse™ Bone Graft kit components; (C) the LT-CAGE device; and (D) procedure for combination at the point of use. (*Copyright Medtronic. LT-CAGE Incorporates Technology by Gary K. Michelson*).

with formaldehyde and sterilization using ethylene oxide [17]. This process can be problematic, as endotoxin removal can be an issue with such materials and there have been indeed product recalls by Integra Lifesciences, the manufacturers that perform the sterilization of the scaffolds for Medtronic, due to potential contamination issues. The rhBMP-2 and excipients are lyophilized together and then sterilized using a nanofiltration process. The three components are then combined by the physician at the point of use in a sterile field using aseptic technique before implantation in the patient (Fig. 2.7D). In this way, the manufacturer has avoided trying to identify a suitable terminal sterilization method that would not adversely affect any of the components if they were combined together and provided in a finished form for off-the-shelf usage.

2.2.4 Electronics, bioabsorbables, and other novel materials and the future of combination product development

An article published by Robert Langer almost a decade ago was predictive of the ascendance of the combination product and described the convergence of two or more distinct scientific disciplines as the basis of a new device, process, or product (Fig. 2.8) [18]. The overlapping of advancements in the Biotechnology, Information Technology, and Nanotechnology arena provides opportunity to develop complex novel systems encompassing wide-ranging functions such as microelectrical mechanical systems for sensing drug delivery, high-throughput biology and microarray technology,

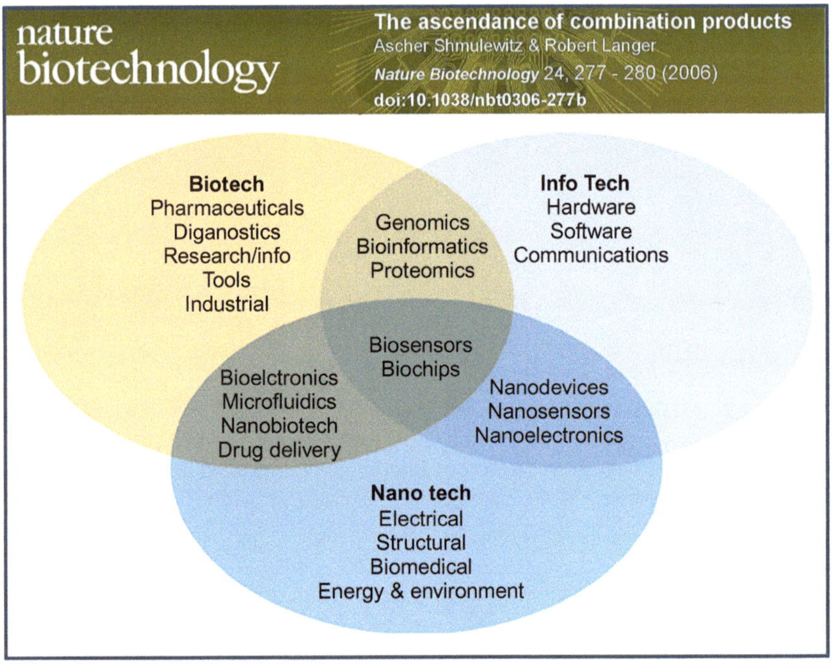

Fig. 2.8 The ascendance of combination products by convergence of technology platforms [18].

new biomaterials for medical devices, novel routes of administration to better target drugs, through to wholly tissue engineered solutions.

Combination products with electrical components have been around for some time, often, as in the case of photodynamic therapy, the drug is provided separately from the electronic device that generates the light that is used to activate it, the two being cross-labeled for use in specific indications. Some newer technologies, however, have integrated electronics and methods to sterilize such products can be challenging. Steam, EtO, chemicals with moisture, and irradiation methods can all adversely affect electronics. The use of low-temperature dry-heat processes (below 160°C) for sterilization has been used for some medical implants and can be suitable for some electronic materials that are heat resistant as long as the new process is adequately qualified and validated. The same goes for novel polymers that would otherwise perish under some of the harsher sterilization conditions. For instance, silicone prostheses are sterilized by dry heat as they undergo radiation-induced cross-linking or retain high levels of ethylene oxide if treated using EtO. Bioabsorbable polymers will degrade by design and processes used to sterilize these materials can accelerate the degradation process if not developed with the appropriate attention to the chemistry (Fig. 2.4). Solutions must therefore be sought, especially as it is predicted that advances in bioresorbable implant technologies will drive further combination product market expansion in the near future. Notable is the acquisition of TYRX Inc. by Medtronic in early 2014. With a recently FDA cleared AIGISRx combination product based on a resorbable antibacterial envelope to reduce surgical site infections associated with cardiac implantable electronic devices, AIGISRx R antibacterial envelope for use with spinal cord stimulators, and Pivitab antibiotic impregnated resorbable hernia mesh in development, Medtronic have signaled a clear investment in bioabsorbable polymer technologies.

And where is all of this heading? The most likely scenario is an ever-increasing degree of product functionality and complexity. A new class of combination products known as 'Multipurpose Prevention Technologies (MPTs)' [19] are under development that are gels, intravaginal rings (IVRs), or barrier devices used with a gel or film that have a combination of contraceptive, microbiocidal, and/or anti-sexually transmitted infection (STI) properties with different mechanisms of action that act to prevent pregnancy, HIV, and/or STIs. For example, novel IVRs that combine contraceptive hormones (e.g., Levonorgestrol) with Tenofovir, a drug shown to prevent both HIV and HSV-2 are being developed. This is just one example of a combination product in which two or more different drug types are combined with a single delivery device in order to address multiple therapeutic indications where targeted locoregional delivery from the device makes sense. Obviously, attention to drug-drug interactions will be important consideration for such products, but again, one of the biggest challenges in their development process will be the identification of an appropriate route to sterilization that maintains individual component integrity.

References

[1] A.L. Lewis, M.R. Dreher, Locoregional drug delivery using image-guided intra-arterial drug eluting bead therapy, J. Control. Release 161 (2) (2012) 338–350.

[2] A.L. Lewis, R.R. Holden, DC bead embolic drug-eluting bead: clinical application in the locoregional treatment of tumours, Expert Opin. Drug Deliv. 8 (2) (2011) 153–169.

[3] A.L. Lewis, et al., DC bead: In vitro characterization of a drug-delivery device for transarterial chemoembolization, J. Vasc. Interv. Radiol. 17 (2) (2006) 335–342. Pt 1.

[4] S. Baltes, et al., Doxorubicin and irinotecan drug-eluting beads for treatment of glioma: a pilot study in a rat model, J. Mater. Sci. Mater. Med. 21 (4) (2010) 1393–1402.

[5] S. Glage, et al., Evaluation of biocompatibility and anti-glioma efficacy of doxorubicin and irinotecan drug-eluting bead suspensions in alginate, Clin. Transl. Oncol. 14 (1) (2012) 50–59.

[6] L.I. Linkow, J.R. Wagner, Management of implant-related problems and infections, J. Oral Implantol. 19 (4) (1993) 321–335.
[7] Printzen, G., Relevance, pathogenicity and virulence of microorganisms in implant related infections. Injury, 1996. 27 Suppl 3: p. SC9–15.
[8] D.G. Allison, A review: taking the sterile out of sterility, J. Appl. Microbiol. 87 (6) (1999) 789–793.
[9] E. Regar, G. Sianos, P.W. Serruys, Stent development and local drug delivery, Br. Med. Bull. 59 (2001) 227–248.
[10] B.J. Lambert, T.A. Mendelson, M.D. Craven, Radiation and ethylene oxide terminal sterilization experiences with drug eluting stent products, AAPS PharmSciTech 12 (4) (2011) 1116–1126.
[11] Y.V. Il'ichev, L. Alquier, Effects of E-BEAM sterilization on drug-eluting stents: Paclitaxel degradation elucidated by LC-MS-MS with information-dependent acquisition, J. Chromatogr. Sci. 49 (10) (2011) 807–817.
[12] J.H. Baron, R.K. Aggrawal, M. Azrin, Development of c7e3 fab (abciximab) eluting stents for local drug delivery: effect of sterilization and storage, Circulation 98 (17) (1998) 4487.
[13] A. Hagan, et al., Preparation and characterisation of vandetanib-eluting radiopaque beads for locoregional treatment of hepatic malignancies, Eur. J. Pharm. Sci. 101 (2017) 22–30.
[14] D. Carugo, et al., Benefits of polidocanol endovenous microfoam (Varithena(R)) compared with physician-compounded foams, Phlebology 31 (4) (2016) 283–295.
[15] R. Scherliess, et al., Induction of protective immunity against H1N1 influenza a(H1N1) pdm09 with spray-dried and electron-beam sterilised vaccines in non-human primates, Vaccine 32 (19) (2014) 2231–2240.
[16] B. McKay, Local sustained delivery of recombinant human bone morphogenetic protein-2 (rhBMP-2), Conf. Proc. IEEE Eng. Med. Biol. Soc. 2009 (2009) 236–237.
[17] W. Friess, et al., Bone regeneration with recombinant human bone morphogenetic protein-2 (rhBMP-2) using absorbable collagen sponges (ACS): Influence of processing on ACS characteristics and formulation, Pharm. Dev. Technol. 4 (3) (1999) 387–396.
[18] A. Shmulewitz, R. Langer, The ascendance of combination products, Nat. Biotechnol. 24 (3) (2006) 277–280.
[19] D.R. Friend, et al., Multipurpose prevention technologies: products in development, Antiviral Res. 100 (Suppl) (2013) S39–S47.

CHAPTER 3

Terminal sterilization

Vu H. Le[a], Scott Weiss[b], Brad Lundahl[c], Stan Lam[d]
[a]Divisional Engineering, Abbott, Temecula, CA, United States
[b]Industrial Microbiology, Johnson & Johnson Microbiological Quality and Sterility Assurance, Raritan, NJ, United States
[c]Johnson & Johnson Microbial Quality and Sterility Assurance, Raritan, NJ, United States
[d]Process and Technology Development, Stryker Neurovascular, Fremont, CA, United States

Contents

3.1 The history of sterilization

Sterilization in the early 20th century was based on the work pioneered in the late 19th century by the likes of L. Pasteur, C. Chamberland, R. Koch, and E. Bergmann, and usually involved high heat processes such as dry or moist heat for medical products made of high heat-resistant materials. Following World War II, a confluence of scientific and technological advancement in the areas of microbiology, medical products, polymer chemistry, and radiation physics, as well as private and public [1,2] investigation of food preservation technologies led to the development of low-temperature terminal sterilization technologies [radiation and ethylene oxide (EO)] in the 1950s based on a probabilistic model of sterility [3].

Today, just over 60 years later, the most commonly used modalities of terminal sterilization processing of medical products are radiation, EO, and

Assurance of Sterility for Sensitive Combination Products and Materials
https://doi.org/10.1016/B978-0-12-805082-8.00003-7

moist heat. The most prevalent technologies—radiation and EO sterilization—comprehensively address the ideal characteristics of a sterilization technology identified by Rutala [4]. The worldwide predominance of these two modalities of terminal sterilization can be attributed to these characteristics, along with readily available proven consensus standards and guidelines [5,6] that were jointly developed by the industry and regulatory bodies addressing every aspect of medical product sterilization [7].

3.1.1 History of radiation sterilization

In 1904, shortly after the discovery of X-rays by W.K. Roentgen (1895) and the observation of radiation emitted by uranium by H. Becquerel (1896), the application of radiation for food preservation was evaluated by S. C. Prescott and W. L. Underwood [8–10]. Interest in the biocidal application of radiation led to the issuance of a UK patent to Appleby and Banks in 1905 for the application of ionizing radiation to kill bacteria in foods. A US patent was later issued to D.C. Gillett in 1918 for an apparatus for preserving organic materials by the use of X-rays [8]. In 1929 preliminary investigational work was published on logarithmic mortality rates of bacteria exposed to radiation by M. Curie [11], F. Holweck [12], and M.A. Lacassagne [13] at De L'Academe Des Sciences in Paris. By the late 1960s, gamma irradiation was commonly used for large-scale terminal sterilization of medical devices due to increased availability of radioactive sources [14, 15] and the higher reliability of gamma irradiators with respect to electron beam accelerators of/at that time.

Sources of radiation used for terminal radiation sterilization supply electrons from electron beam accelerators or photons from either a radioisotope (Co^{60}, Cs^{137}) or accelerators (bremsstrahlung) to transfer energy to the product. Source electrons or photons ionize molecules and atoms of the product material initiating a cascade of scattered electrons throughout the irradiated product. These scattered electrons damage nucleic acids, proteins, and enzymes essential for a microorganism's growth and proliferation [16]. The penetrating ability of these radiation sources facilitate the sterilization of bulk medical products in their final packaging (terminal sterilization).

The amount of energy transferred and absorbed by a product is measured in units of absorbed dose called kilograys (kGy). The absorbed dose is measured with a dosimeter and calibrated dosimetry system [17–19]. Sterility resulting from a validated radiation sterilization process is based on a bioburden method [20] that directly correlates the minimum absorbed dose received by the product to a sterility assurance level (SAL).

Thus, product release after radiation terminal sterilization processing relies neither on a test for sterility [21] nor on the assay of a biological indicator (BI) [22] for product release. Product approval is based on parametric release (dosimetric release); a declaration that the product is sterile based on records demonstrating that the process parameters (absorbed dose) were delivered within the specified range [23].

3.1.2 History of EO sterilization

EO was first isolated in 1859 by the French chemist Charles-Adolphe Wurtz and by the early 20th century it was being used as a fumigant for insects. In the late 1920s, Llyod A. Hall identified a vacuum process using EO gas to sterilize spices used in packaged meats. This was shown to prevent premature spoilage of meats caused by the bacteria in the seasoning spices.

The EO terminal sterilization process exposes product surfaces to gaseous EO. It is a powerful alkylating agent that reacts and denatures nucleic acid and proteins resulting in nonviable microorganisms. EO is a highly effective surface sterilant but, because it does not penetrate, it requires gaseous contact of all surfaces for it to be effective. Product and product packaging intended to be EO sterilized must be permeable to heat, humidity, air, and EO [6].

The critical process parameters that impact lethality of EO are as follows:

(a) concentration of EO
(b) temperature of the product prior to and during exposure to EO
(c) pressure/vacuum conditions affecting product load uptake of EO[a]
(d) humidity in terms of steam impacting the product uptake of EO[1]
(e) packaging and product that impact diffusion of EO to the surfaces
(f) time during which specified thresholds of parameters ‘a’ through ‘e’ occur

Unlike radiation sterilization, multiple process parameters must be controlled and monitored throughout each phase of the EO sterilization process. In addition to sterility, other critical factors typically evaluated in the validation are residuals [24] and endotoxins [25]. The sterilization process must also demonstrate EO, ethylene glycol (EG), and ethylene chlorohydrin (EC) residuals as well as endotoxins must be proven to be below regulated thresholds levels. Although the EO sterilization process is typically validated, monitored, and product is released with BIs [22], parametric monitoring and release can also be used [6].

[a]Note: pressure/vacuum/packaging/product does not directly affect the lethality. However, it does affect the movement of EO and moisture into product load, thereby affecting the efficacy of EO process lethality.

3.1.3 History of dry and moist heat sterilization

The use of both dry and moist heat to preserve food has been alluded to since biblical times, though it was more magic than science. In Exodus XVI 16:23 and 24, Moses instructed "So bake what you want to bake and boil what you want to boil. Save whatever is left and keep it until the morning." "So they saved it until the morning, as Moses commanded, and it did not stink or get maggots in it." Later in Roman times, physicians would boil their instruments before treating the gladiators. In 1830, William Henry applied scientific methods to devise a jacketed hot air sterilizer and demonstrated that heat could disinfect cholera infected clothing. Although it was recognized that the prognosis of patients improved when the medical instruments were first heat treated, it took the convergence of discovery and technology to really initiate the fundamental understanding of heat sterilization as we know it today. The concept of linking microbes to disease and the subsequent development of the pasteurization process by Louis Pasteur in 1862 was key in the evolution of the technology. Later, another key discovery was the development of the intermittent heating process to inactivate heat-resistant bacteria by John Tyndall in 1876. The technology that enabled this originated from the food industry. In 1795 Nicholas Appert invented canning as a means to preserve food and in 1860 Denis Papin invented the pressure cooker. Louis Pasteurs' pupil Charles Chamberland developed the first pressure steam sterilizer (autoclave) in 1876 and Ernst von Bergmann, a German physician, put it all together in 1885 when he steam sterilized surgical dressings. Around this time, Robert Koch developed a silk thread impregnated with anthrax spores to investigate the various sterilization methodologies. He demonstrated that moist heat was much more efficient than dry heat at inactivating the bacteria and was able to define the exact conditions required. In 1885, Gaston Poupinel developed a dry heat sterilizer which was adopted by many hospitals in France. Another milestone that enabled the validation of the sterilization process was achieved in 1891 by Fred Kilmer who developed BIs. As the technology continued to improve, the approaches to standardize the sterilization process followed. In the same year, Ernst Von Bergmann began heat sterilization of surgical instruments.

In the early 1980s, the Parenteral Drug Association published its technical report on sterilization validation [PDA Validation of Moist Heat Sterilization Processes: Cycle Design, Development, Qualification and Ongoing Control (1980, revised 2007), PDA Validation of Dry Heat Processes Used for Depyrogenation and Sterilization (1981, revised 2013)] followed by the International Standards Organization with their standards in the 1990s. Both moist and dry heat rely on the same fundamental mechanism to inactivate microorganisms. The thermal energy results in the denaturation of proteins and enzymes. This loss of functionality of enzymes causes the death of the organism. The difference in the efficiency between dry and moist heat arises from the difference in efficiency with which the thermal energy is transmitted to the organism. In dry heat, the energy is transmitted by the conduction of heat through air. This is relatively inefficient. Moist heat sterilizations rely on the high latent heat of vaporization to efficiently transfer heat from the steam to the microbes to affect the kill. As the saturated steam interacts with the surface, it condenses, transferring the heat to the surface. The change in phase from gas to liquid also results in a reduction in volume which in turn draws more gas to the surface. This process continues until the surface equilibrates in temperature with the steam. As this energy interacts with the organism, it rapidly raises the temperature of the cell. This denatures the proteins, enzymes, and DNA. The denaturation of the enzymes results in the loss of function and death of the organism. Key factors which govern both dry and moist heat sterilization are as follows:

Factor	Dry	Moist
Barriers	Thermal	Thermal and tortuosity path
Temperature	Of oven	Of Steam
Pressure	No	Yes
Time	Yes	Yes

3.2 Sterile validation of current methods

The risk of non-sterile product reaching the patient is extremely low, but the criticality is high because many of the device combination products are parenteral or implantable. Even if the probability of the event happening is very low, the impact can be catastrophic. The paradox for sterility testing is that the low incident rate and the destructive nature of the testing make the verification strategies impractical. The validation of a terminal sterilization process requires qualification of the product, the equipment, and the process. The definition of packaging constraints, microbial quantity, and quality of the product are all needed to meet the rigor of validation. In contrast to aseptic processing, the validation of the terminal sterilization process provides a specific SAL for the product. Terminally sterilized devices usually eliminate the need for product tests for sterility since the validation of the process provides a higher confidence level of product sterility than product sterility testing. The major sterilization processes of EO, radiation, and moist heat have well-developed standards and will be discussed to provide an insight into the validation of other novel sterilization methodologies.

3.2.1 Product qualification

Product specifications and associated processes of sterilization must be defined before moving into the validation of a terminal sterilization process. Material compatibility and ranges of conditions in the sterilization process must be understood to select the terminal sterilization method for a combination product. For example, radiation creates free radicals and cross-linking that can be destructive to things such as an active ingredient or the device itself. Similarly, EO reacts with materials and can change the performance of an active ingredients or device. For these reasons, maximum conditions—that is, maximum dose or maximum temperatures and concentrations—for product functionality must be determined. Minimum process conditions that could impact the effectiveness of inactivating microbes are addressed through the validation of the sterilization process—or the ability of the process to render the product sterile.

3.2.2 Equipment qualification

The qualification of the equipment used to deliver the sterilization process is typically broken into two categories: installation qualification and operational qualification. Installation qualification allows for a documented review of equipment location, utilities required, safety, instrumentation and calibration, and proper operation of the equipment and ancillary systems. Operational qualification documents must show that the system (equipment, ancillary equipment, controls) can deliver the required process within defined tolerances. The operational qualification is usually executed after the process has been defined, and the installation and operational qualifications can be executed without product loading as the qualifications are focused on equipment operation and performance.

3.2.3 Sterilization validation approaches

Microbial validation of the terminal sterilization process determines the minimum conditions required to render the product free of viable organisms. Since it is impossible to prove absolute sterility, the terminal sterilization industry has defined this as an SAL. The SAL is defined as "the probability of a single microorganism occurring on an item after sterilization." [1] It has been demonstrated that the SAL or viability or survival versus sterilization treatment follows a log-linear relationship. The SAL of the product is the relationship between the amount of sterilization treatment and the starting population and resistance of the microbial challenge to the sterilization process is shown in Fig. 3.1.

An important characteristic of this chart is the D-value which is the exposure required to achieve inactivation of 90% of a population of the test organism under stated conditions. The D-value is a measure of resistance the challenge presents to the sterilization process. Understanding the D-value of the product's bioburden through the process allows for extrapolation of time and conditions required to deliver the specified SAL for the product.

The product bioburden is a critical process input for terminal sterilization validation. Bioburden is defined as "the population of viable microorganisms on or in the product and/or sterile barrier." [23] An understanding of the product bioburden is required to understand the sterilization process and possible validation approach. The combination of the product, packaging, and quantity and types of microorganisms on the product present the challenge to the sterilization process. Collectively, these contribute to the resistance of the microbial population to the sterilization process. The estimates of the bioburden as well as its susceptibility to the sterilization conditions need to be characterized.

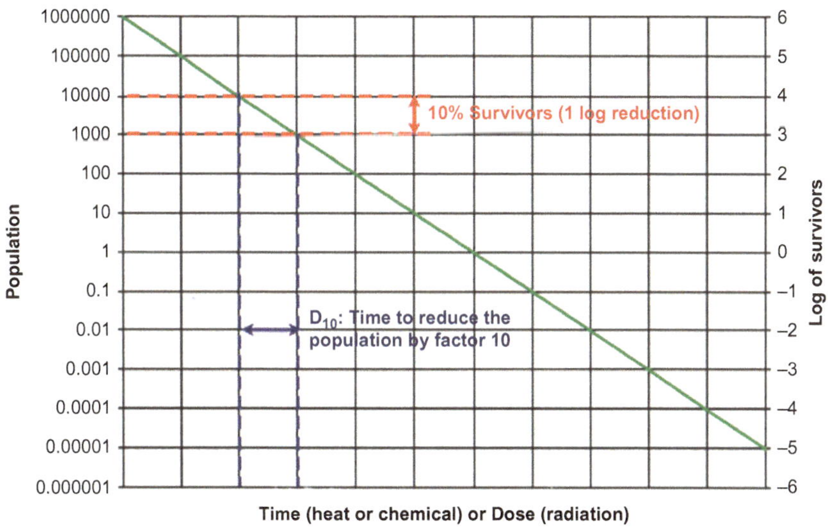

Fig. 3.1 SAL plot.

A relationship between the product configuration and microorganisms presented to the sterilization process helps define the approach for validation. In all sterilization modalities, product test of sterility is conducted at conditions less than the routine sterilization process to establish characteristics such as the D-value. The validation of the terminal sterilization process utilizes this information to include safety factors to extrapolate to the desired SAL. The test **of** sterility, performed as part of development, validation, or requalification, should not be confused with the test **for** sterility. The test **for** sterility examines microbial growth following routine processing (aseptic or sterilization). A test for sterility cannot, inherently, extrapolate to an SAL as the test for sterility can only indicate a sterile or non-sterile article [26].

There are three approaches to validate the terminal sterilization process:

1. Bioburden-based approach,
2. Bioburden and BI-based approach, and
3. Biological indicator approach (overkill)

3.2.3.1 Bioburden-based approach

The bioburden-based approach to terminal sterilization validation focuses on the normal microbial flora on the product and can lead to the development of terminal sterilization processes more gentle or appropriate for combination products. All validation methodologies for radiation sterilization—Methods 1, 2A, 2B, and VD_{max}^{SD}—are based on the bioburden approach. The bioburden-based approach may also be used for gas and heat sterilization processes (ISO 11137-2:2012, ISO 11135-1: 2014, ISO 14937:2009, and ISO 17665-1:2006).

The bioburden-based approach is executed using unsterilized product samples that have been manufactured in accordance with routine production—this allows for challenging the microbial flora resulting from the process and materials, as opposed to samples prepared in a manner different from the routine manufacturing process. The product samples are typically exposed to subprocess conditions of the terminal sterilization process. In radiation, samples are processed at a low verification dose or at increasing doses, with samples from each tested for sterility. In EO and other gas-based processes, samples could be processed at different exposure times, maintaining constant humidity and gas concentration, or concentrations can be varied keeping all other variables constant, or some other combination of variation. For moist heat, since time is most easily and precisely controlled, the product is exposed at full temperature for different times while maintaining the other cycle conditions, such as heat up, temperature, and cool down. The intent is to determine the resistance level the normal microbial flora present on the product and packaging has to the sterilization process.

By knowing the bioburden population (count) and relative resistance of that population from the subprocess studies, an extrapolation can be made as to the final processing conditions required to deliver the required SAL.

A terminal sterilization process established using the bioburden-based approach is sensitive to changes in microbial population and resistance. For this reason, a robust bioburden monitoring program should be implemented with routine sterilization process checks. In radiation, routine sterilization process checks are accomplished through the dose audit process. The dose audit involves exposing product samples to a dose selected based on the bioburden or established in the incremental studies, which is referred to as the verification dose. The verification dose is based on the expected resistance of the bioburden population to deliver an SAL of 10^{-1} or 10^{-2} (based on the method used to establish verification dose). The samples are then submitted for tests of sterility, with the results either supporting continued effectiveness of the overall sterilization process or indicating that investigation is required into the validity of the sterilization dose. Similarly, an EO process validated with the bioburden-based approach should include routine monitoring of the effectiveness of the sterilization process by exposing the product samples to fractional process conditions with subsequent product sterility testing. Heat sterilized product with the bioburden-based approach (probability of survival approach) should include routine presterilization bioburden monitoring to ensure that there has not been a shift in bioburden level or microbial resistance to temperature. The monitoring of key equipment and process parameters should also be conducted routinely for all sterilization processes.

3.2.3.2 Bioburden and BI-based approach

The bioburden and biological indicator approach introduces a surrogate BI to validate and routinely monitor the process for EO sterilization. Radiation validation does not use BIs and focuses only on the bioburden-based approach.

As with the bioburden-based approach, the bioburden and BI-based approach requires strong knowledge and control of the product bioburden. Bioburden fluctuations could have a significant impact on the effectiveness of the validated sterilization process. The bioburden recovery method and frequency of monitoring should be effective at detecting shifts in the microbial flora.

The bioburden and BI-based approach establishes a resistance profile of the product bioburden against a BI. The BI is composed of a homogenous population of an organism with a known resistance to the sterilization process being validated. *Bacillus atrophaeus* is commonly used for EO sterilization, while *Geobacillus stearothermophilus* is used for moist heat. The BI is typically selected with a population equal to or slightly greater than the product bioburden. Product samples and BIs are exposed to graduated conditions and sterility tested to establish the resistance profiles between the two populations. Once the comparative resistance is known, the validation of the sterilization process can be executed with only the BI.

The bioburden and BI-based approach introduces the concept of a process challenge device (PCD), defined as an "item designed to constitute a defined resistance to a sterilization process and used to assess performance of the process." [5] As previously discussed, the resistance of the product to the sterilization process involves the product configuration, packaging, and the types and quantities of organisms present. While validating the sterilization process with only the product bioburden, product configuration challenges are inherent in the process—meaning the microbial flora and the location on/in the device have already been considered in the validation approach (bioburden-based approach). When using a surrogate BI, the difficulty of getting the sterilant to all locations in the device should be challenged. This leads to the development of the PCD. An evaluation of the product configuration and the packaging should determine where the PCD/BI should be placed to create the greatest challenge to the sterilization process. The comparative resistance of the BI and the bioburden should account for the use of the PCD—the BI is placed in the most challenging location to sterilize.

The PCD may be generated by inoculating the actual product in difficult to reach locations, or may be composed of a surrogate device that presents an equal or greater challenge to sterilize as the product and associated bioburden. Again, this is accomplished through product tests of sterility following exposure to reduced, or fractional, conditions.

Once the PCD and the comparative resistance between the PCD and bioburden are understood, the validation of the sterilization process is executed using only the PCD. The PCD is exposed to incremental conditions to establish the D-value. Once the D-value is understood, the exposure conditions can be extrapolated to determine the final cycle conditions required to deliver the specified SAL.

3.2.3.3 BI approach

The third method for validating a terminal sterilization process is the BI approach, also known as the overkill method. This method uses a BI challenge to validate the sterilization process, like the combined BI/bioburden-based approach. Unlike the combination approach, the overkill method uses a high population of resistance organisms on the BI. This extreme population of highly resistant organisms will result in actual SALs in excess of the desired SAL.

A relationship between the product bioburden and the PCD must be established such that the PCD presents a greater challenge to the sterilization process. In many cases, the population of the BI used in the PCD is several logs greater than the product bioburden (e.g., 10^6 vs 10 [3]). The comparative resistance is established by exposing the PCD and product samples to a fractional sterilization process, where both are tested for sterility. In this study, as the PCD must be more resistant than the product samples, all product samples must be negative for growth and some portion of the PCD samples should be positive for growth from the sterility test results.

After the PCD is proven to be more resistant to the sterilization process than the bioburden, the validation of the sterilization process begins. The PCD is exposed to conditions where all PCD challenges are negative for growth. Once this endpoint is found, the exposure time (typically) is multiplied accordingly (typically doubled) to reach the required SAL. Again, this approach is very conservative and will result in a sterilization process that far exceeds the required conditions needed for the product SAL. The sensitivity of product components and active ingredients adds challenges to using the overkill approach for validation.

3.2.4 Validation overview

Terminal sterilization inactivates microorganisms as opposed to aseptic processing which involves preventing contamination of sterile materials. The validation of the sterilization process starts with understanding the impact of the sterilization modality to the product performance, at the highest sterilization conditions, as well as the ability to inactivate the microbial organisms at the lowest conditions. Because of this fundamental difference, and inherent safety factors therein, regulatory agencies prefer terminal sterilization process evaluation before the use of aseptic processing whenever possible [27].

There are multiple modalities for terminally sterilizing products. The selection of the modality is based on the compatibility of the device with a process. Materials react differently to the modality chosen. Sensitive combination devices should not only focus on material compatibility, but also on how things such as the active ingredients react during sterilization and the shelf life of the product after sterilization.

There are multiple approaches to the validation of a terminal sterilization process: bioburden-based approach, bioburden and BI-based approach, and biological indicator approach (overkill). All three methodologies are based on understanding the impact of the sterilant on the microbial bioburden or surrogate. All three methods tend to overestimate the SAL because of inherent safety factors that are added to the method. The relative safety factor tends to increase, going from the bioburden-based approach to the bioburden and BI-based approach to the BI approach. These approaches developed for radiation, EO, and dry/moist heat sterilization can be applied to other sterilization modalities.

3.3 Future approaches to sterilization

There is a growing number of products that are submitted to the Food and Drug Administration (FDA) that utilize sterilization processes beyond the traditional methods, which are referred to as established methods given the history and longtime acceptability. The FDA guidance considers these new sterilization technologies to be novel methods [28]. Established sterilization methods have a history of being applied to many products and understanding of effects on materials. They are divided into two categories: A and B. Category A includes methods with a long history such as radiation, EO, and dry/moist heat. Category B includes methods that are newer but still have precedence with the methods being applied to products, such as hydrogen peroxide, ozone, and flexible bag EO systems. Novel methods such as vaporized peracetic acid, microwave radiation, sound waves, and ultraviolet light, have very limited data.

Established methods have worked successfully with typical materials found in single-use medical device products and will likely continue to do so in the future. With continuing innovations in electronics, materials, diagnostics, controlled and targeted delivery as well as active ingredients (particularly biologics) the limitations of the established methods are becoming apparent. The complexities of sensitive combination products have introduced new material compatibility challenges. The current simple devices are tolerant to the sterilant and processing conditions optimized for these devices, but this might no longer be adequate for more sensitive devices.

These processes are being pushed to their limits in order to tighten ranges as more innovative devices are being developed. Combination products increase the challenge further as different product functions often have different tolerances to the sterilization modalities. For example, a sensitive drug with an electronic medical device will have increased stability issues with both EO and radiation sterilization.

Established terminal sterilization methods may not be compatible with new products. Alternative gas sterilization technologies provide an additional tool to terminally sterilize innovative products. These technologies will be referred to as alternative gas methods as opposed to the established EO gas methods. The vendors of these alternative gas methods have taken a similar approach as established methods to characterize effects on materials. AAMI TIR 17:2008[35] expanded the scope of material evaluations to include radiation, EO, moist heat (steam), dry heat, hydrogen peroxide, and ozone.

The alternative gas methods follow a similar sterilization validation methodology as EO, with the general requirements detailed in ISO 14937: 2009 [29]. The physical sterilization processes are different from EO because of the nature of the three novel gases, for example, nitrogen dioxide, vaporized hydrogen peroxide, and vaporized peracetic acid. All these gasses have the ability to operate at ambient conditions with temperature ranging between 18 and 30 °C. Although humidity typically ranges between 30% and 100% for standard cycles, vaporized peracetic acid has the ability to sterilize as low as 16%. As with any process, there are tradeoffs. As the dwell time decreases, the relative humidity must increase to provide the microbial kill. The standard full-length cycle of the alternative gasses is much shorter, typically under 4 h. The cycle time for most of these alternative gasses is much shorter than EO because the gasses and their breakdown products are much less toxic than the carcinogenic EO.

The mechanism of gas delivery has changed dramatically. Rather than an extended injection and dwell commonly used for EO, alternative gasses are exposed to the product in multiple short pulses of specific duration and dwell time. The gases are evacuated and exchanged with air between pulses resulting in dramatically shorter product contact time. The unique properties of the gases, in combination with the dramatically lower exposure times, result in an expanded list of compatible materials to screen during the development of the product.

Exploitation of the unique properties of novel gasses may enable the sterilization of new products. An example of this is the terminal sterilization of pre-filled syringes. Sterilization gas with low permeability could enable the sterilization of surfaces and components of the final package without penetrating the pre-filled content. Another example is the sterilization of bioabsorbable polymers which can be compromised when treated using the established methods but has been demonstrated to have good compatibility with alternative gases. Radiation sterilization of these polymers at traditionally high doses causes degradation, while the high temperature and high relative humidity of EO processing can lower the T_g and plasticization of the materials, which can result in the softening as well as the loss of the secondary and tertiary structure [30]. The degradation or softening of the material reduces structural integrity and the performance of devices such as stents or bone screws.

Another opportunity might involve combining novel methods with established methods to create an adjunct sterilization process. Consider the scenario of a combination device composed of a drug-coated polymer which has a limited sterilization dose range due to degradation from a radiation process. The reduction of bioburden can be achieved through improved controls in the manufacturing process which would enable validation of a lower sterilization dose. Typically in a combination product, only certain components of the drug-device combination product are sensitive to the sterilant. The application of novel gas sterilization treatment during the manufacturing process just prior to the incorporation of the sensitive component provides extra insurance against incidental spikes in bioburden that could occur during earlier stages of the manufacturing process.

The final example is the rapidly expanding consumer wearable sector. The merging of technology and health care has created the digital health space which is transforming chronic care management between the patient and the physician. The FDA is actively engaged in this sector as it brings several benefits such as personalized medicine, increased compliance, and reduced costs to the patients [31]. This next wave of innovation introduces electronics to the already complex matrix of polymers, metals, and drugs in the existing sensitive combination devices. New sterilization methods and new validation approaches are a welcome addition providing an additional toolset to the engineer to bring products to the market.

3.4 Conclusion

The early development of what is now the established sterilization modalities occurred when devices were constructed with simpler materials and designs. These devices are extremely tolerant to the assaults of radiation, EO gas, and dry/moist heat, allowing robust sterilization cycles to be developed. An in-depth understanding of microbial loading along with microbial response to the sterilant resulted in conservative cycles that produced safe products. Innovative new products are pushing current sterilization technology to the limits, as developers are challenged to address new materials, and new drugs with complex designs. These advances are pushing the sterilization technology to new limits. As developers continue to innovate in areas such as controlled drug delivery, sensitive combination product that provide multiple benefits, and the incorporation of electronics into devices, the sterilization technology and validation strategies will have to be as innovative to match the needs of these devices.

References

[1] R.A. Molins, Food Irradiation: Principles and Applications, Wiley & Sons, May 24, 2001, (ISBN: 0-471-35634-4).

[2] D. M. Boyd, An Evaluation of Radiation-Processed Foods for Military Rations, Defense Technical Information Center Compilation Part Notice ADP014623.

[3] ANSI/AAMI ST67:2011 (R2017), Sterilization of Health Care Products—Requirements and Guidance for Selecting a Sterility Assurance Level (SAL) for Product Labeled Sterile.

[4] W. Rutala, D.J. Weber, CDC Guidance for Disinfection and Sterilization in Healthcare Facilities, HICPAC, 2008.

[5] ISO 11137-1 Sterilization of Health Care Products-Radiation-Part 1: Requirements for Development, Validation, and Routine Control of a Sterilization Process for Medical Devices.

[6] BS EN ISO 11135-1:2014 Sterilization of Healthcare Products-Ethylene Oxide-Requirements for Development, Validation and Routine Control of a Sterilization Process for Medical Devices (ISO 11135:2014).

[7] J. Broad, L. Nawrocki, Making Sure its Sterile, Medical Design, July 1, 2006.

[8] M. Karel, D. B. Lund, Physical Principles of Food Preservation, CRC Press, (June 20, 2003, ISBN:0824755790).

[9] J.F. Diehl, Safety of Irradiated Foods, CRC Press, Karlsruhe Germany, ISBN, Dec 1, 1999, pp. 0–8247-93447.

[10] Institute Archives, M.I.T. Libraries, December, https://libraries.mit.edu/mithistory/research/schools-and-departments/school-of-science/department-of-biology/, 1995.

[11] M. Curie, Sur l'etude des courbes de probabilite relatives a l'action des rayons X sur les bacilles, Compt. rend. Aca. Paris 188 (1929) 202.

[12] M.F. Holweck, Production de rayons X monochromatiquies de grand longueur d'onde. Action quantique sur les microbes, Compt. rend. Aca. Paris 188 (1929) 197.

[13] M.A. Lacassagne, Action des rayons X de grande longueur d'onde sur les microbes. Establissement de statistiques precises de la mortalite des bacteries irradiees, Compt. rend. Aca. Paris 188 (1929) 200.

[14] Sister Mary Andre Chorzempa, Ionizing Radiation and its Chemical Effects: A Historical Study of Chemical Dosimetry (1902–1962), Oregon State University, June 1971.

[15] J. Silverman, Radiation processing: The industrial applications of radiation chemistry, J. Chem Ed 58 (1981) 168–173, https://doi.org/10.1021/ed058p168.

[16] K. Suzuik (Ed.), Vol. 4, in: Selected Papers in Biochemistry, Radiation Biology of Microorganisms, University Press, Baltimore, London, Tokyo, 1971.
[17] ISO/ASTM 52628, Standard Practice for Dosimetry in Radiation Processing, ASTM International, West Conshohocken, PA, 2013, p. 2013.
[18] ISO/IEC 17025:2005, General Requirements for the Competence of Testing and Calibration Laboratories.
[19] 21CRF 820.72 Title 21, Chapter I – Food and Drug Administration, Department of Health and Human Services, Subchapter H-Medical Devices, Part 820, Subpart G – Production and Process Controls, Inspection, measuring, and test equipment.
[20] ISO 11137-2 Sterilization of Health Care Products-Radiation-Part 2: Establishing the Sterilization Dose.
[21] United States Pharmacopeia National Formulary (USP40-NF35) 2017, Sterility Tests <71>.
[22] ANSI/AAMI/ISO 11138-1:2017, Sterilization of Health Care Products-Biological Indicators-Part1: General Requirements.
[23] ANSI/AAMI/ISO TIR11139:2006, Sterilization of Health Care Products—Vocabulary.
[24] ISO 10993-7: 2008 Biologic evaluation of medical devices-Part 7: Ethylene oxide sterilization residuals.
[25] ANSI/AAMI ST72:2011 Bacterial Endotoxins-Test Methods, Routine Monitoring, and Alternatives to Batch Testing.
[26] E. Daniell, T. Bryans, K. Darnell, J. Hansen, V.M. Hutchins, M. Saavedra, Product Sterility Testing… to Test or Not to Test? That Is the Question, in: Industrial Sterilization, Sep 2016.
[27] B. Lambert, T. Mendelson, M.D. Craven, Radiation and ethylene oxide terminal sterilization experiences with drug eluting stents, AAPS PharmSciTech 12 (4) (Dec 2011).
[28] https://www.fda.gov/downloads/MedicalDevices/.../ucm109897.pdf.
[29] AAMI TIR 17: 2008, Compatibility of materials subject to sterilization.
[30] https://www.ncbi.nlm.nih.gov/pmc/articles/PMC3225553/.
[31] https://www.fda.gov/medicaldevices/digitalhealth/.

Further reading

[32] Guidance for Industry and FDA Staff, Current Good Manufacturing Practice Requirements for Combination Products, US Department of Health and Human Services, Food and Drug Administration, Office of Combination Products (OCP) in the Office of the Commissioner, Center for Biologics Evaluation and Research (CBER), Center for Drug Evaluation and Research (CDER), Center for Devices and Radiological Health (CDRH), Office of Regulatory Affairs (ORA), Final Guidance, January 2017.
[33] B.J. Lambert, T.A. Mendelson, M.D. Craven, Radiation and ethylene oxide terminal sterilization experiences with drug eluting stent Products, AAPS PharmSciTech 12 (4) (2011) 1116–1126, https://doi.org/10.1208/s12249-011-9644-8.
[34] B.J. Parsons, Sterilization of drug-device combination products, in: A. Lewis (Ed.), Drug-device Combination Products, Woodhead, Cambridge, 2010, pp. 395–435.
[35] B.J. Parsons, Sterilization of healthcare products by ionizing radiation: Sterilization of drug-device products and tissue allografts, in: S. Lerouge, A. Simmons (Eds.), Sterilization of Biomaterials and Medical Devices, Woodhead, Oxford, Cambridge, Philadelphia, New Delhi, 2012, pp. 212–234.
[36] ISO 14937:2009, Sterilization of health care products — General requirements for characterization of a sterilizing agent and the development, validation and routine control of a sterilization process for medical devices.

CHAPTER 4
Aseptic processing

Hal Baseman
Valsource Inc., Jupiter, FL, United States

Contents

Assurance of Sterility for Sensitive Combination Products and Materials
https://doi.org/10.1016/B978-0-12-805082-8.00004-9

4.1 Aseptic processing of sterile combination products

Combination products are therapeutic or diagnostic products that combine drugs, devices, and/or biological products [1]. They are defined as *two or more separate products packaged together in a single package or as a unit and comprised of drug and device products, device and biological products, or biological and drug products* [2]. Sterile combination products have the additional requirement that the final product must be sterile. Sterile combination products are a growing and important segment of health-care therapies.

There are the US and international regulatory documents associated with the manufacture of combination products. The FDA has published guidance on both combination products as well as aseptic processing. The FDA 2004 Guidance on Aseptic Processing outlines the expectations for the manufacture of sterile drug products using aseptic processing. The GMPS for combination product is a merger of relevant sections of CFR Parts 210, 211, and 820 [3]. The European Union has recently revised its Annex 1 for the manufacture of Sterile Medicinal Products including those using aseptic processing [4].

Manufacturers of sterile combination products are required to comply with all relevant regulations applicable to all parts of the combined product. In general, Drug GMPs are more prescriptive than Device GMPs, while Device GMPs are more system focused. For the most part, the same GMPs and rules for aseptic processing apply to the sterile drug part of the combination product as do for any sterile drug product. While regulatory requirements and in some cases, terminology may be different, the expectations for aseptic processing are the same. Therefore, with respect to the requirements and expectations of aseptic processing, if a company follows the Drug GMPs and guidance, that manufacturer is probably covering what it will need from an aseptic processing perceptive. If the manufacturer follows the Device GMPs and guidance, additional requirements are likely needed to document device design controls, supplier controls, CAPA, management controls for devices, design history, control over the device and the drug in a combination product, risk analysis for the entire product, and interaction of the drug and device.

4.2 Drug product sterility

Drug product sterility can be achieved by terminal sterilization of a sealed/packaged product, aseptic processing, or a combination of these two methods. A key difference between sterilization and aseptic processing is the former actively seeks to destroy all viable microorganisms from the product while the latter attempts to prevent product contamination by carefully controlling the conditions and actions designed prior to sealing, completion, and final packaging.

Another strategy is to combine aseptic processing and sterilization. Here aseptic processing principles and methods are used to reduce the bioburden or level of microbiological contamination in the product to very low levels and a final sterilization treatment is employed to increase the level of sterility assurance. This is sometimes referred to as post-aseptic lethal treatment.

This chapter will primarily focus on aseptic processing of the drug product part of the combination product. The chapter will not present all aspects or requirements for aseptic processing but will discuss some of the points to consider for manufacturing sterile combination products using aseptic processing.

Where all parts of the combination product can be terminally sterilized, it is required that they be. However, not all components or products can withstand terminal sterilization. Components may lose functionality and product may lose potency or purity because of exposure to heat, radiation, or other methods of sterilization. When one or more of the components or products of a combination product cannot be terminally sterilized, aseptic processing is typically used for that part or the entire combination product. There are three options for manufacturing a sterile combination product using aseptic processing:

1. Manufacture and assemble all components—drug, device, and packaging aseptically.
2. Manufacture and assemble some of the components aseptically and then assemble with sterilized components.
3. Manufacture and assemble all components aseptically and subject product to post-aseptic lethal or decontamination treatment.

4.3 Aseptic processing

Aseptic processing is a set of process steps, conditions, and actions taken to render product and components sterile and prevent microbiological contamination of that product and those components prior to final assembly and sealing. The Parenteral Drug Association (PDA) Technical Report 22, Process Simulations for Aseptically Filled Products, defines aseptic processing as the handling of sterile materials in a controlled environment in which the air supply, facility, materials, equipment, and personnel are regulated to control microbial and particulate contamination to acceptable levels and the process for manufacturing sterile products by which microbiological contamination is eliminated from the product and product contact surfaces protecting the product from sources of contamination [5, 6]. The US FDA and European EMA define asepsis, as the aseptic state, is the state of control attained by using an aseptic work area and performing activities in a manner that precludes microbiological contamination of the exposed sterile product, with aseptic defined as something that is free from contamination caused by harmful bacteria, viruses, or other microorganisms [Internet] [3, 4].

Each of these definitions places an emphasis on prevention of microbial exposure through the design and implementation of a microbiological contamination control strategy. Whereas terminal sterilization establishes sterility assurance levels (SAL) or probability of non-sterile units (PNSU) surviving the sterilization process, aseptic processing establishes a level of confidence or an assurance of sterility through the prevention and control of contamination.

There are useful regulatory, health authority, and industry guidance documents that present expectations for aseptic processing control strategies, including the US FDA Aseptic Processing Guidance (2004), The European Union Annex 1 GMPs for Sterile Medicinal Product Manufacturing (2008 with draft revision 2017), and the Parenteral Drug Association (PDA) Aseptic Processing Points to Consider Parts 1 and 2 [3, 4, 7]. Despite these guidance documents, aseptic processing in practice can be one of the more challenging methods for manufacturing sterile drug product.

There are several reasons for the difficulty in manufacturing sterile products using aseptic processing. Prevention of contamination might be more advantageous for a product than active processes such as sterilization, but it is generally more difficult to accomplish and prove that it was done successfully. The following are some of the reasons aseptic processing can be challenging.

The metric for success is not well defined. In a moist heat termination sterilization process, we are actively eliminating microorganisms through physical destruction of those microorganisms. To accomplish this, the amount of energy needed to destroy the level of microbial contamination is determined. The amount of heat and duration of heat exposure under predetermined conditions needed to destroy the microorganisms can be both calculated and measured and confirmed experimentally thus providing ample evidence that the microorganisms have all been destroyed. In the case of aseptic processing, we are preventing the action of contamination. The complexities of proving a negative, or the lack of existence of microbes, are more challenging than proving a positive.

Detection of contamination or sterility is difficult. Nondestructive detection of microbes is difficult and, in many cases, not feasible. Sterility testing (USP <71>) is destructive and therefore requires a limited sampling number. The current sampling and testing practice do not result in a statistically relevant assurance of sterility. Environmental monitoring of clean room air and surfaces is imperfect, with significant variability in results and capability to obtain meaningful results. Environmental contaminant recovery and testing might not be complete and sample sizes and locations are often limited due to probe placement and instrumentation. In addition, environmental monitoring material placement can involve significant and, in some cases, risky human intervention into critical aseptic processing areas.

There is a lack of observable correlations. Current approaches to aseptic process control do not provide a means to measure sterility assurance in aseptic processing. The correlation between the observed and the desired (or undesired) outcome is relatively poor. Air profile (smoke) studies, differential pressures, air velocity, first air principles, ascending and descending clean room classifications, and aseptic technique are designed to prevent microorganisms from contacting and contaminating sterile surfaces or contents. These methods are not surrogates for an indication of contamination. In other words, we do not know for certain the level of disruption in these controls is needed to contaminate the contents of a container.

Aseptic processing involves significant variables. Aseptic processing is complex. It involves the interplay between environment, microorganisms, contamination vectors, complicated manufacturing methods, and human behavior. Human behavior is variable and unpredictable. Training, monitoring, performance feedback, coaching, supervision, observation, human factor consideration, ergonomic process design, barriers, and automation can only help reduce variability and the effect of variability but never eliminate the inherent variability of human performance. Therefore, any process that depends on human intervention and activity will be inherently variable.

The impact of the failure is severe. Failure of the aseptic process can result in contamination of the sterile product and could impact patients significantly. Not all microbial contamination observed in the environment, on personnel, or on product contact surfaces will result in microbiological contamination of the product and not all microbiological contamination of the product will result in patient health issues. However, because the product is typically implanted or injected, the patient risk profile is similar between the various microbial sources. This makes the controls for all levels of contamination a high concern.

Based on the standard definition of process risk where risk is the relationship of severity of a hazard (in this case loss of sterility), probability of the hazard occurring, and ability to detect the hazard, the severity would be high, occurrence inconclusive, and detection relatively poor. Therefore, the overall risk is high.

Because the current detection technology and the correlation between what can be observed, and the desired outcome is not strong, significantly reducing this risk through detection is not likely. The best way to control an aseptic process failure and reduce the aseptic processing risk is by reducing the likelihood of occurrence through sound risk and science-based process control strategies and design.

4.4 Aseptic process design

Proper design and planning of the aseptic process are essential to ensuring a compliant and effective sterile combination product manufacturing process. One of the first steps is to understand the objective of the process and its relationship to product quality and output. The objective of the aseptic process is preventing contamination during the manufacturing of the product.

4.5 Sterility by design

To provide effective process control, it is essential to identify all process variables that impact the product output. Attaining primary confidence in the process should happen during the design of the process, rather than during final process qualification testing or continued process verification. It is this confidence that enables the company to commit to the process design [8].

4.6 Line of sight [9]

One method of identifying critical process parameters early in the development stages is to use the line of sight (LOS) approach, as noted in Fig. 4.1. In a LOS approach, the objective of the aseptic process design is kept in sight. All actions are focused on achieving this objective. The objective is the establishment and maintenance of a critical quality attribute (CQA), in this case, product sterility. All actions taken in the design should be able to

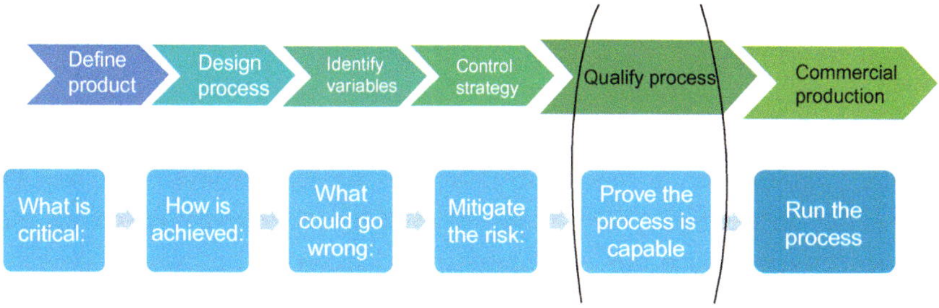

Fig. 4.1 Line of sight process control approach.

be linked to meeting this objective and ultimately, all objectives should be addressed by one or more aspects of the process design.

The LOS approach to process control and validation can be described in six progressive steps.

1. The first step identifies the critical quality attributes of the product. These are the conditions and functions that define the product as safe and efficacious. These attributes might include specifications for strength/potency, safety/sterility, purity, identity, and functionality. Where possible, it is important that these attributes be stated as quantified, measurable criteria or specifications. This will help in designing process control strategies and actions, and in determining process qualification tests and acceptance criteria.
2. The second step determines the process steps needed to achieve the quality attributes. Each quality attribute relies on one or more processes to achieve that attribute. For example, sterility might involve clean room, sterilization of components, sterilization of product, sterilization of filler parts, assembly of sterilized filler parts, holding of sterile materials, transport of components, and sealed containers.
3. The third step identifies variables that might be inherent in the process that could result in loss of, or pose a risk to, the quality attributes. This might include operator error, poor process design, failure of sterilization processes, nonintegral packaging or container integrity, environmental contamination, etc.
4. The fourth step determines the controls or control strategy needed to mitigate the risks. At the end of this step, the company should have the understanding and confidence in the process and associated controls to finalize the design and install the systems needed to perform the process. This might include gowning qualification, environmental monitoring, clean room disinfection, load pattern, and recording of sterilization

cycles, design of sterilization circuit, container integrity inspection and testing, and process monitoring.

5. The fifth step develops the means to test if the control measures are effective in addressing process variability and risk. This might be considered where *traditional* installation/operational qualification and process performance qualification studies occur. Once step five is complete, the company will have the documented evidence that the process can deliver product that meets critical to quality attributes with reliability and capability and be confident that it is ready to begin commercial manufacturing. This might include design and installation qualification of clean room, HVAC system, critical utilities, operational qualification of filling lines, and aseptic process simulations.
6. The sixth step occurs during commercial manufacturing. It involves the continued or ongoing acquisition and evaluation of a subset of information obtained from performing the process during manufacturing. This step is designed to monitor the process to assure that the process is maintained in a qualified state. This enables additional variables that have not been previously uncovered or adequately controlled to be identified and additional controls to be implemented to address these new variables to improve the control of the process. This might include environmental monitoring, process performance metrics (e.g., process capability), statistical process control charting, process failures, investigations, OOS results, sterility failures, and audits [9].

Control strategies and process steps designed to mitigate one risk may add additional risks to other product attributes. The interaction of process steps could pose a risk to the quality of the product. These unintended consequences should be considered during the process design. For example, the use of a more aggressive disinfectant and sanitization program might be a control strategy for reducing the risk of environmental contamination but may also damage filling equipment or pose a risk of chemical contamination to product. In this case, it would be important not only to address the intended benefit of the mitigation action but also to address the potential unintended consequence of the action.

4.7 Defining aseptic process requirements

The manufacturing of sterile combination drug products will involve several key steps. These steps will depend on the objectives of the manufacturing operation, as reflected in the desired outcome of the process or the production needs of the operation. This would include the type of products and therapies, annual production output required, rate of output, number of products, global regulatory requirements, flexibility and redundancy business strategy, cost strategy, and production timing.

The quality aspects of the product might be contained in a quality target product profile (QTPP). The QTPP is a prospective summary of the quality characteristics of a drug product that ideally will be achieved to ensure the desired quality, considering the safety and efficacy of the drug product [10, 11].

The business objectives of the production process must also be known. This information is often noted in what is referred to as a project charter. The project charter includes such information as:

- annual or periodic production quantities,
- critical quality attributes of the product,
- supply chain considerations, and
- patent or approval timing issues.

A useful tool to capture and summarize the aseptic processing strategy is the LOS Evaluation Table (Table 4.1). This tool links the quality attributes as defined to the process steps and identifies how the process will be controlled, monitored, and documented.

4.8 Basis of design

The basis of design defines the limitations and requirements to meet the objectives of the manufacturing operation and process. These limitations and requirements may be driven by questions related to technical, regulatory, market, cost, safety, business, or other concerns and circumstances. For example:

- Is the product inherently sterile or can it be sterilized by filtration or by some other means?
- Is the product sensitive to air, light, or temperature?
- Can the product be sheared or damaged through the filling process?
- Will the product react to manufacturing and fill system materials of construction, such as metals, stainless steel, plastics, etc.?
- Must the product be lyophilized for functionality or stability?
- Does the product involve autologous and allogeneic cell collection?
- Does the product have special or unusual holding, storage, collection, or transport requirements?
- Is the product hazardous, hypoallergenic, or requires containment considerations?

Table 4.1 Example of line of sight process evaluation.

CQA	Process steps	Process variables	Control strategies	Qualification/validation testing
Safety—sterility	Sterilization	Inadequate temperature and exposure time, air in system, steam conditions, incorrect or random loading patterns, excessive bioburden, incorrect components	Autoclave design, cycle monitoring/recording, established loading patterns, automated receipt and storage of components, clean component and ingredient storage conditions, properly sized filters, training, first air principles, smoke studies	Autoclave IOQ, temperature mapping, BI studies, air removal studies
Safety—sterility	Aseptic processing	Poor aseptic and gowning technique	Clean room design, clean room sanitization, airflow, workflow, people flow …	Air profile studies, risk assessment, training, disinfectant efficacy studies, environmental and personnel monitoring, gowning and personnel qualification aseptic process simulations
Safety—sterility	Container closure integrity	Leakage	Container/closure design, sealing process control, leakage inspection systems	Design qualification, vendor audit, incoming inspection, leak detection studies and testing, in process testing

- In what jurisdictions and markets will the product be distributed?
- What are the cost limitations?
- Are there unusual stability limitations (e.g., temperature, humidity)?
- Will product be produced in an existing facility, and if so, then—what are the limitations of that facility?
- Will redundant manufacturing systems be required?

The product requirements, along with contamination control and efficiency strategies will influence technology decisions. As such, the answers to these questions will in part determine the technologies and methods used to manufacture the products, including the use of:

- aseptic or terminal sterilization processes,
- batch or continuous process manufacturing,
- manual fill systems,
- conventional semiautomated filling systems,
- barrier systems such as Isolators, RABS (restricted access barrier systems), or Blow Fill Seal and Form Fill Seal,
- robotics and automated filling systems,
- steam/sterilize in Place product filtration and transfer systems, and
- continuous total particulate and/or viable environmental monitoring systems.

The outcome of this evaluation will help provide the information contained in column 2 of Table 4.1.

4.9 User requirement specification (URS)

The URS is important for process design because it sets the criteria for process performance based on product quality requirements. The URS is developed once the basic technology strategy is set. The URS presents more specific user needs that can be translated into a manufacturing process design. The URS should be prepared prior to the design of the process and the selection of systems. The URS can then be used to develop the strategy to select and define critical aspects of the process, process parameters, and qualification/validation acceptance criteria. Information and design requirements from the URS can then be used during a design qualification and process qualification to ensure that the critical aspects of the process have been incorporated. The URS should address anticipated process variables that might adversely affect the sterility of the product and control strategy to ensure reliable process performance and output meeting production/product requirements. The URS can be used to obtain information needed to complete columns 2 and 3 of the LOS Evaluation table (Table 4.1) [12].

4.10 Aseptic practices

The sterile drug product aseptic manufacturing process includes steps that expose surfaces or materials to potential sources of microbiological contamination. These sources can include people, the environment, equipment or facility surfaces, utilities, gases, water, or raw material inputs such as components, parts, ingredients, other materials, etc. The protection of the sterile product and product contact surfaces is essential to the reliable performance of the aseptic process and is the objective of good aseptic practices. This objective should be captured in the validation approach.

Monitoring and detecting contamination could be easy, as might be the case with bioburden of materials, or difficult, as might be the case with environmental contamination. Sporadic or intermittent contamination, as might be the case with biofilm, or human intervention-related contamination tends to be particularly challenging.

Aseptic practices are designed to protect the product from microbiological contamination and include controls such as:

- Clean room design and operation
  - smooth and cleanable clean room surfaces to reduce the potential for contamination in seams and openings;
  - clean room equipment design to allow for accessibility and workflow;
  - clean room equipment cleanable surfaces;
  - positioning of equipment and functions with minimal first air interference;
  - clean room high-efficiency particulate air (HEPA) filtered air supply with adequate velocity,
  - clean room differential air pressure for correct flow from clean to less clean areas;
  - clean room HVAC temperature and humidity controls to minimize operator discomfort, particulate static charge, and microbiological growth;
  - clean room air changes to remove contaminated air;
  - design of adjacent clean room spaces and areas to allow for work and personnel flow and protect cleaner areas; and
  - work, personnel, equipment, materials, and component flow to reduce the risk of contamination of cleaner areas and materials from contact with less clean items;
- Material/product preparation and handling
  - sterilization and decontamination of product contact materials and surfaces;

    - wrapping, holding, and assembly of sterilized product contact parts;
    - wrapping, holding, and transfer of sterilized components, and containers;
    - holding and transfer of sterilized product;
    - sanitization materials entering the clean room areas;
    - product sterilization and transfer;
    - product container closure integrity;
    - attachment of lines, filters, tanks, vessels, hosing, etc.
    - pre-sterilization solution compounding;
    - cleaning, sanitization, and sterilization of takes, vessels, filters, and lines;
    - cleaning, sterilization, and depyrogenation of components;
    - cleaning and sterilization of parts;
    - sterilization or filtration of product;
    - container closure sealing and integrity; and
    - inspection of filled units.
- Aseptic processing activities
    - inherent and corrective interventions;
    - environmental monitoring practices and techniques;
    - environmental monitoring sampling plans;
    - clean room personnel supervision and observation;
    - aseptic technique and first air principles;
    - clean room personnel rest periods, breaks, fatigue, ergonomic process design;
    - personnel personal hygiene and illness recognition;
    - clean room gowning and personnel monitoring;
    - reporting of discrepancies and deviations; and
    - exclusion or restriction of materials, personnel, items, and such from clean room.

These process steps and actions are essential in the holistic approach to aseptic process validation. All equipment supporting the process should be qualified and each process should be validated.

4.11 Interventions and activities in the aseptic processing critical area

Interventions usually are human activities or manipulations that occur during the aseptic process in the proximity to product contact surfaces. This poses a risk to product quality especially aseptic process performance. In general, because people represent a significant source of bioburden, human manipulations or interventions should be minimized. Where interventions are necessary, steps should be taken to minimize the risk of product contamination from such actions. Interventions can be categorized as inherent (routine) or corrective (nonroutine).

Inherent interventions are manipulations in the critical aseptic processing area that are part of the process. They must be performed for the process to proceed. These interventions include activities such as setting up of the filler parts, installing filters, loading components, placing environmental monitoring sensors, removing fill checks, and transferring materials.

Corrective interventions are activities that might occur but do not have to occur. These include such activities as removing of fallen vials, removing of jammed stoppers, clearing of broken containers, adjustments, and minor repair and replacement of parts.

All inherent and corrective interventions should be performed using proper aseptic technique, respecting first air and airflow principles. For corrective interventions, additional steps may be required to reduce contamination risk and reestablish aseptic conditions after the performance of corrective interventions. These steps can be determined through a risk assessment and may include such actions as removal of open containers in near the intervention, disinfection of the area where the intervention is performed, additional environmental monitoring, and/or segregation of post-intervention product [5, 7].

4.12 First air principles

One of the most effective control measures for the prevention of microbiological contamination is the use of clean airflow. Aseptic practices are those process steps and related functions performed using aseptic techniques that adhere to first air principles in a protected classified environment. First air refers to an uninterrupted HEPA filtered air source traveling to the sterile entity. The good aseptic technique involves observing first air principles and avoids placing potentially contaminated objects in between the source of HEPA filtered air and the sterile entity (product or product contact surface). Interventions using sterilized objects that are handled correctly, such as sterilized forceps that disrupt first air have a low risk of contaminating the sterile product. Interventions using non-sterile objects, such as gloved hands or gown sleeves that disrupt first air have a higher risk of contaminating the sterile product. The risk can be mitigated by designing the process or positioning the activity so that the airflows from the HEPA filter to the sterile entity without the air interacting with the potentially contaminated object (see illustration in Fig. 4.2).

Aseptic practices rely, on clean air surrounding the sterile product and product contact surfaces, directed airflow, good process design, clean surfaces, and proper aseptic technique. The qualification of aseptic practices should address all variables that could adversely affect sterility. For example; the variables associated with clean areas might include the capability and integrity of HEPA filters, differential pressure, and air changes. The variables associated with directed airflow might include unidirectional airflow, air velocity, interference, and turbulence. The variables associated with process design might include ergonomics, equipment design, operator access, and barriers. The variables associated with clean surfaces might include porous surfaces, seams, reaction to cleaning materials, and limited access. Finally, variables associated with aseptic technique might include gowning, training, access, excessive exposure, and obstacles.

First air includes air above the working surface. The air below the working surface, for example below the operator's waist, is generally considered to be non-sterile. If the operator's gloves fall below their waist it assumed that the gloves are contaminated and must be changed or disinfected with a proven disinfectant solution (e.g., sterile filtered 70% IPA).

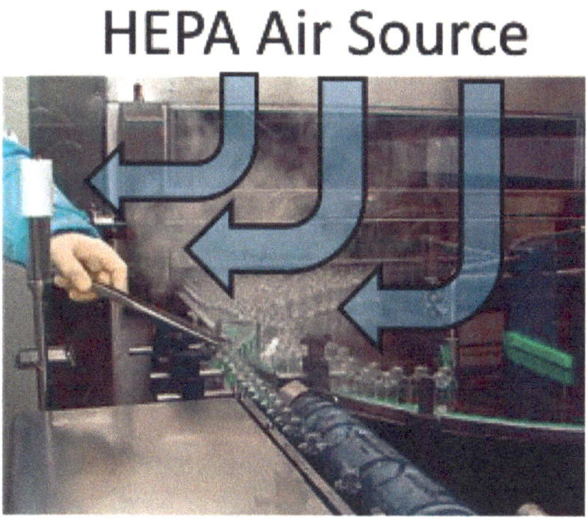

Fig. 4.2 First airflow. *(Courtesy of ivtnetwork.com)*

4.13 Environmental monitoring

The environment can be a significant potential source of bioburden. The proper design, operation, and performance of the clean room are essential to the control contamination. Trending the environmental monitoring data essential indication of clean room is kept in control. Risk-based approach should be used to determine methods, locations, and frequency of monitoring. The FDA Aseptic Processing Guidance, the EU annex 1 GMPs, and ISO Standard 14644–1 and 2, as well as many other global health authority guidance and regulations, set requirements, and expectations for environmental monitoring [3, 7, 13, 14].

Environmental monitoring is an indicator that the clean room is controlled and remains in a qualified state. The use of environmental monitoring is challenging because of the limited correlation between the condition of the environment and the sterility of the product. Environmental monitoring should be used as one of the indicators if changes in the environment have occurred since the process had been qualified. In this case, the evaluation of environmental monitoring trends is more useful than evaluating excursions from prescribed limits.

Environmental monitoring sample locations and sampling frequencies should be selected on a risk basis considering conditions that might impact product sterility as well as predict excursions. Locations within critical filling and product contact exposure areas should be monitored to detect immediate system failures or sources of contamination. Locations in adjacent areas with lower classification can be useful indicators of systemic changes or predictions of contamination in critical cleaner areas. Risk-based approaches that consider workflow, material and personnel traffic, equipment operation, and critical exposure of product would be particularly useful.

Environmental monitoring for viable contamination is typically achieved using passive settling plates, active air sampling devices—both stationary and portable, swabs and contact plates. The environmental monitoring method should be appropriate for the surface being monitored. Active air samplers and settling plates can be used for air quality. Contact plates can be used for smooth, relatively flat surfaces, such as stopper bowls, walls, and machine bases. Swabs can be used for smaller surfaces or surfaces with crevices, such as filling needles and stopper tracks.

Environmental monitoring, especially total (also referred to as nonviable) particle monitoring where possible should be continuous and automated. There should be minimal mechanical systems located in the critical space. Manipulations and interventions associated with the monitoring in the critical area should be minimized as well.

When environmental monitoring cannot be continuous or automated, such as when the placement of plates or swabs in a critical area, the activity is considered an intervention. Care and proper aseptic technique should be taken to the place of materials or related environmental monitoring activities such as contact plates and swabs on product contact parts or surfaces. When possible, it is preferable to execute tasks at the end of the aseptic process or fill to avoid contaminating those parts or surfaces. Personnel performing environmental monitoring may be quality, microbiology, or operations personnel provided they are properly trained and supervised [7, 15].

Recovery rates for microorganisms/colonies can be variable, and this fact should be considered when evaluating results. Monitoring that requires personnel to intervene, such as swabs and contact plates, will increase variability. This variability and these recovery rates should be determined and considered when analyzing and reporting results.

Excursions from prescribed limits or levels, as well as upward trends, should be investigated. These excursions may not necessarily be the result of system failure. The location, level, type of contamination, seasonal variation, activities occurring during the monitoring, and the impact on product quality should be considered when deciding process and product disposition associated with from an excursion.

4.14 Personnel monitoring

Clean room operators, monitoring personnel, mechanics, and other clean room personnel represent both a significant source and a risk of microbial contamination. Personnel should be qualified to enter and perform their functions in the clean room. Personnel qualification includes training, testing, and ongoing monitoring.

Personnel monitoring should be performed at prescribed intervals through the aseptic process. The monitoring may include finger impression plates for gloves, contact plates or swabs for gowns and other surfaces. Personnel monitoring after gowning may be part of an overall gowning qualification or continued verification of gowning technique.

Scheduled and random monitoring of gloves and gowns should be employed, including personnel monitoring upon exit from clean room or prior to re-gowning should be performed. Monitoring of gloves through finger impression plating should be performed prior to removal of gloves, prior to changing of gloves and upon exit from the cleanroom, and after certain more extensive or critical interventions. Ample time from sanitization of gloves to the monitoring of gloves should be considered, that is, the monitoring of gloves should not be performed on gloves that have been recently sanitized. Gown monitoring locations should be selected based on potential risk posed to the sterile product. Typically, higher risk areas on the gown such as seams, openings or connections are present as well as sleeves, front, and neck area should be monitored.

Personnel monitoring may be performed by quality, microbiology, or operations personnel providing they have the proper training and supervision. Personnel monitoring should be performed in an area where it does not pose a risk to aseptic process operations.

4.15 Clean room design

The use of clean rooms represents a significant contamination control method. Clean rooms should be designed to be cleaned and sanitized using commercial disinfectants. Seams, cracks, crevices, and openings where dirt and contamination can collect but cannot be adequately cleaned or sanitized should either be eliminated or sealed. Walls, floors, ceilings, doors, and other surfaces should be smooth and cleanable. Drains should not be present in areas where critical aseptic operations are taking place. Access to clean rooms should be limited to clean personnel and materials. The use of interlocking doors and active air pass-throughs that limit cross contamination between clean materials and personnel with soiled or compromised materials and personnel should be used. Access to clean rooms should be through controlled areas using proper technique to decontaminate materials, transfer carts, equipment, and other items.

Clean rooms should be supplied with HEPA filters with the filter(s) positioned to adequately cover and protect critical operations. Initially, clean rooms should be classified and HEPA filters certified to meet certain air cleanliness and performance standards such as ISO Standard 14644 [13, 14]. Clean rooms should be qualified at rest and in operation to confirm that they maintain classification during operation. HEPA filters should be certified to confirm they are integral and perform properly. HEPA filters and clean rooms should be recertified and re-qualified on a periodic basis to ensure that they perform at a qualified state and level.

Clean rooms should have adequate air supply to maintain proper differential pressure between areas of higher cleanliness and lower cleanliness. Air supply should be sufficient to prevent the accumulation of contamination from material transfer, personnel activities, and other operations. Airflow should be established according to those levels of activity. HEPA air velocity should be sufficient to prevent contamination at working surfaces near and around exposed products and product contact surfaces.

Clean room conditions such as temperature and humidity should be controlled to ensure operator comfort, reduce risk of particulate contamination through static charged from dry air, and reduce risk of microbiological contamination from higher temperatures and humidity.

Clean rooms are specified by the EU as Grade A through D and by the US FDA as ISO 5 through 7 as presented in Table 4.2. These designations reflect expectations for total particulates and viable contamination. The most critical aseptic operations and activities are performed in Grade A and ISO 5 areas, with lower grade areas used for support functions.

4.16 Airflow or air profile visualization (smoke) studies

An important tool in designing and confirming proper clean room airflow in clean room and critical aseptic processing areas are air visualization studies. These are sometimes referred to as air profile or smoke studies. These studies involve the application of a visual medium in the form of a mist that enables the visualization of the flow of air. Typically, gaseous liquid nitrogen is used to visualize airflow, but other means can be used. Caution should be exercised in the selection of visualization material and method to ensure that the method is safe for personnel and equipment.

Air visualization enables the confirmation that

(a) filtered airflows from cleaner areas to less clean areas in a manner that would sweep contamination from clean surfaces toward exhausts,

(b) airflows from areas of higher differential pressure to areas of lower differential pressure, and.

(c) little or no turbulence is present at clean area surfaces.

Air visualization studies can be used to help plan and design the placement of equipment and components, and it can also be used to help train clean room operators by showing the effects of proper and improper aseptic technique (Fig. 4.3).

Table 4.2 Comparison of clean room designations [15].

Particle size	ISO 14644	US FDA (Aseptic Processing Guidance)	USP <1116>	EU Annex 1 and WHO	Japan (Aseptic Processing Guidance)	JP XVI
	Clean room standards—airborne particulate limits (particles/m^3)					
	ISO 5	**ISO 5/Class 100**[a,b]	**ISO 5/Class 100**	**Grade A Grade B (at rest)**	**Grade A Grade B (at rest)**	**Grade A Grade B (at rest)**
≥0.5 μm	3520	3520[c]	3520	3500	3520	3520
≥5 μm	29	Not specified	Not specified	1[d]	20[c]	Not specified
	ISO 6	**ISO 6/Class 1000**	**ISO 6/Class 1000**	**NA**	**NA**	**NA**
≥0.5 μm	35,200	35,200	35,200	NA	NA	NA
≥5 μm	290	Not specified	Not specified	NA	NA	NA
	ISO 7	**ISO 7/Class 10,000**	**ISO 7/Class 10,000**	**Grade B (operation) Grade C (at rest)**	**Grade B (operation) Grade C (at rest)**	**Grade B (operation) Grade C (at rest)**
≥0.5 μm	352,000	352,000	352,000	350,000	352,000	352,000
≥5 μm	2900	Not specified	Not specified	2000	2900	Not specified
	ISO 8	**Class 100,000**	**ISO 8/Class 100,000**	**Grade C(operation) Grade D (at rest)**[e]	**Grade C (operation) Grade D (at rest)**	**Grade C(operation) Grade D (at rest)**
≥0.5 μm	3520,000	3520,000	3520,000	3500,000	3520,000	3520,000
≥5 μm	29,000	Not specified	Not specified	20,000	29,000	Not specified

[a]Class 100 and Grade A are defined as requiring unidirectional flow by all applicable guidelines.
[b]Obsolete US Federal Standard 209E classification added for continuity.
[c]Class titles for US FDA and USP indicate equivalent particle counts per ft.
[d]ISO 4.8 based on reduced limit for particles ≥5 μm.
[e]Grade D operational particulate counts are dependent on the operation and are not defined by any guideline.

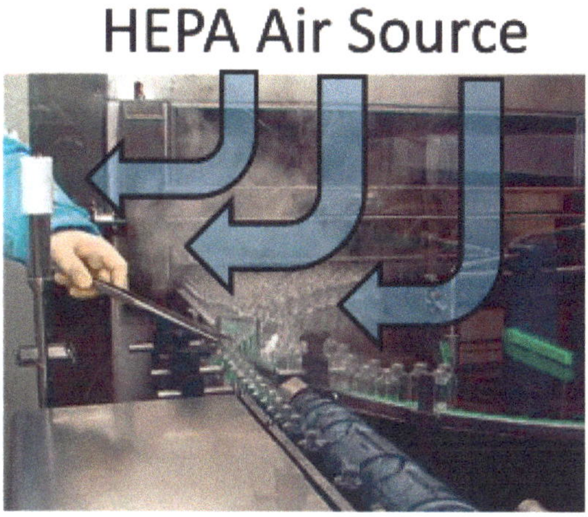

Fig. 4.3 Smoke in airflow profile study. *(Courtesy of ivtnetwork.com)*

4.17 Isolators, RABS, BFS, and other advanced aseptic barrier systems

The use of barrier systems to protect sterilized product and product contact surfaces from the environment and personnel is an effective means to prevent microbiological contamination.

Isolators or barrier isolators are generally closed or partially closed systems containing component handling, conveying, filling, and sealing systems. Isolators are typically decontaminated using gases such as vapor phase hydrogen peroxide, peracetic acid, or other chemical means. Access in and out of isolators is strictly controlled. Isolators are not opened during operation, and personnel access is limited through decontaminated glove ports. The access through glove ports enables the reduction of gowning requirements for personnel. Environmental monitoring takes place within the isolators in a similar manner as would be the case with non-isolator open systems. The interior of Isolators is typically designed to be Grade A or ISO 5 and the Isolator itself may be placed in a less controlled area—Grade C or D.

RABS (restricted access barrier systems) are partially closed systems, where the interior is designed to be Grade A or ISO 5 and the RABS is placed in a Grade B area. Personnel access the interior through decontaminated glove ports; however, personnel are typically gowned. The interior of the RABS may be disinfected with a chemical wipe down or decontaminated through fumigation. Restricted access means that there should be no access during aseptic operations.

The design of the manufacturing equipment should consider first air principles. In this example illustrated in Fig. 4.4, the operator must be careful not to reach over the conveying system and open vials to place environmental monitoring plates on the line.

BFS (blow fill seal) is a means to manufacture sterile products in plastic containers. BFS systems are self-contained, continuous manufacturing systems that heat and extrude plastic to form a container, fill, and seal the container in one continuous operation. Typically, BFS lines are in Grade C areas, with the critical areas contained in Grade A or ISO 5 air shrouds or encasements. Operators are typically fully gowned. Environmental monitoring is limited by the size of the shrouded areas, but generally, the same monitoring should occur in or around the critical areas. BFS lines are divided into two types—shuttle and rotary systems. Shuttle systems have open parisons (plastic used to form the container) and parison transport systems. Rotary lines have closed parison systems, where the filler is not exposed to the environment.

4.18 Critical utilities

Compressed gases, nitrogen, compressed air, clean steam, process water, cooling water, vacuum, and power should enter the clean room through sealed systems designed to minimize contamination. Utilities and materials

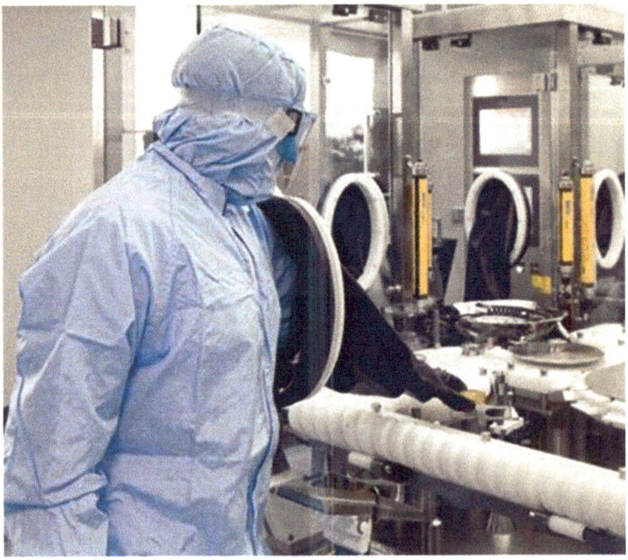

Fig. 4.4 Design for Manufacturing: Importance of environmental monitoring plate location

transporting utilities should, where possible, be treated to eliminate contamination. Compressed gases, nitrogen, and air should be filtered to remove microbiological contamination. Electrical power should be uninterrupted. It is recommended that backup systems be in place to ensure that critical control operations such as airflow through the HEPA system are not interrupted. Routine monitoring and testing of the utilities and materials should be performed to confirm the output of the utilities and quality process materials.

4.19 Aseptic process qualification and validation

The validation of the aseptic process is a holistic approach, encompassing the qualification of all process steps and procedures that may affect product sterility. The FDA Process Validation Guidance and the EU Annex 15 describe a three steps progression for validation of processes. These steps include process design, process qualification, and ongoing or continuous process verification (Fig. 4.5). All critical operations and process steps should be validated, including the cleaning and sanitization of clean rooms and equipment surfaces, the capability of product filters to remove microbiological contamination, equipment operation, formulation, sterilization of product contact surfaces, and aseptic practices [16, 17].

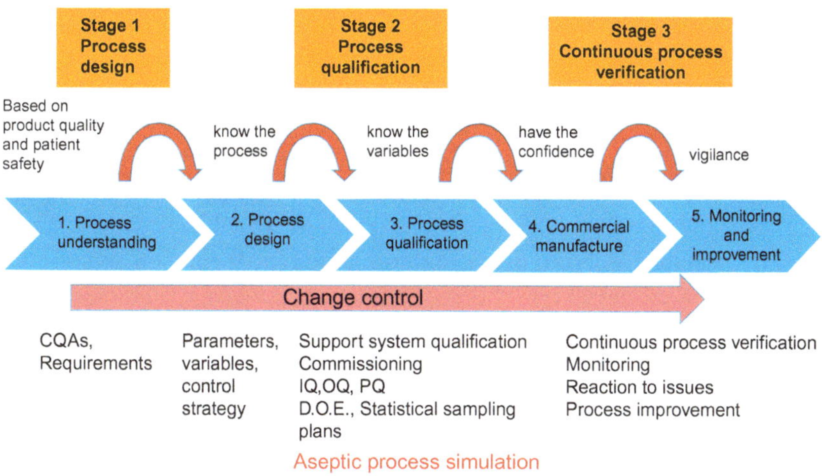

Fig. 4.5 Process validation lifecycle.

4.20 Aseptic process simulation design

Aseptic process simulations are part of the overall aseptic process validation. Aseptic process simulations provide confidence that the aseptic process was designed and performed properly. Aseptic process simulations are but one tool used to validate the aseptic process. Other qualification and validation studies might include:

- microbial retentive capability of the sterilizing filter,
- clean room classification, certification, and qualification,
- clean room disinfectant efficacy studies,
- airflow profile and visualization studies,
- filling and sealing equipment qualification,
- sterilization of product contact parts, utensils, containers, and closures,
- depyrogenaton of containers and closures
- visual inspection of filled units
- container closure integrity studies

Aseptic process simulations, sometimes referred to as media fills, are studies conducted on the aseptic filling process.[a] The aseptic process is simulated or run as close to the actual production procedure as possible except the product is replaced with growth media. The growth media is selected to act as closely to the product properties as practical and still support and indicate relatively low levels of microbial contamination. If there are flaws or weakness in the process resulting in product contamination, then the contamination will likely be discovered in a growth supporting media.

As noted earlier in the chapter, one of the reasons aseptic processes are difficult to validate is trying to prove something has not happened. Filling media in place of product is an attempt to challenge the process and find process weakness. Passing the aseptic process simulation is essentially a failure to find weakness in the process, which proves, in part, the validity of the aseptic process. Conducting multiple aseptic process simulations will increase the likelihood of uncovering process flaws, weakness, or variables.

Part of the overall process validation approach is challenging the capability of the aseptic process to produce sterile products. Aseptic process simulations are a useful tool to confirm the aseptic process design. The simulations

[a]Aseptic Process simulations and media fills are not the same. All media fills, for the most part, are aseptic process simulations. But not all aseptic process simulations are media fills. Media fills involve the filling of media into product containers. Aseptic process simulations often involve such fills, but can also involve bulk compounding simulations, where no fill is performed.

may also uncover unaddressed process variables and weaknesses missed in earlier evaluations. They are a check on the accuracy and effectiveness of assumptions. Process simulations are not a substitute for good process design and should not be relied upon to be the primary judge of the effectiveness of the aseptic process. Confidence in the aseptic process is primarily gained through proper design of the aseptic process with aseptic process simulations being used as for a tool to confirming the acceptability of the process or uncovering missed process variables and weaknesses.

As stated in PDA TR 22, the aseptic process simulations are designed to:

- evaluate capabilities of aseptic processing operation,
- simulate the aseptic process from the point of sterilization to closure of the container, substituting a microbiological growth medium for the sterile product,
- assess changes made to an aseptic processing operation which might impact the sterility of the final product,
- identify weaknesses in aseptic processing which might contribute to the microbiological contamination of the product,
- valuate proficiency of aseptic processing personnel,
- comply with current Good Manufacturing Practice requirements, and
- demonstrate appropriateness of operating practices used in support of aseptic processing.

Solely running aseptic process simulations will not:

- *Validate the aseptic process:* The validation of the aseptic process involves a holistic approach, incorporating validation and qualification of numerous aspects of process design and contamination control.
- *Assure process control*: Process control is assured through careful evaluation of the critical quality attributes, process steps, process variables, risks, and control strategies to mitigate those risks.
- *Determine sterility assurance level*: SAL (sterility assurance level) or PNSU (probability of non-sterile unit), such as those referenced in sterilization processes, cannot be calculated or predicted for aseptic processing by the outcome of aseptic process simulations, due to lack of statistical correlations between observed parameters and desired outcome. In aseptic process simulations, each fill is considered as a separate study with a separate set of conditions. Combining those results to fit a statistical model would not be accurate.
- *Qualify clean room personnel*: Participation in successful aseptic process simulations will not be enough to provide assurance that clean room personnel are properly trained and capable of performing assigned tasks.

- *Qualify support processes and systems*: There are more effective ways to validate support processes, such as wrapping or sterilization of sterilized filler parts, holding conditions for sterile materials, or sterilizing capability of in-line filters, than inclusion in aseptic process simulations.
- *Qualify poor aseptic technique or practices:* Aseptic process simulations should not be used to attempt to qualify a poorly designed or poorly performed aseptic process. If the aseptic process simulation passes, that should not mean that such a process step is acceptable.
- *Train personnel:* Untrained personnel should not participate in aseptic process simulations designed to "qualify" the aseptic process. Trained personnel are a means to eliminate (or reduce) the variability of personnel. In other words, if the aseptic process simulation fails, and the operators were not trained, then those investigating the failure would not know if the failure was due to a process flaw or an operator error.
- *Shakedown an unqualified filling operation*: Using unqualified systems or equipment in an aseptic process simulation should be avoided for two reasons. (1) If the aseptic process simulation fails, and the line was not qualified, then those investigating the failure would not know if the failure was due to a process flaw or an equipment issue, and (2) if the aseptic process simulation passes, and the line qualification is performed later, then any changes which may occur on the line because of the equipment qualification would not be captured in the simulation and therefore that simulation study may not be valid [5].

4.21 Microbial contamination case study

To illustrate the importance of understanding the limitation of the aseptic process simulation test capabilities, consider the case of the qualification of the new aseptic filling operation. The filling process involved the use of an autoclaved, sterilized holding vessel stored for a period in a Grade C environment. To validate the holding of the sterilized vessel, the vessel was held and used in a series of aseptic process simulations. The initial aseptic process simulations passed but failed 6 months later during a periodic requalification (Fig. 4.6).

The source of the contamination was found to be from the contact of environmental microorganisms in the Grade C environment with material used to wrap the open ends of the sterile vessel. The material became wet, and an ineffective barrier because of condensation forming during the storage of the vessel. While this appeared to be a logical explanation for

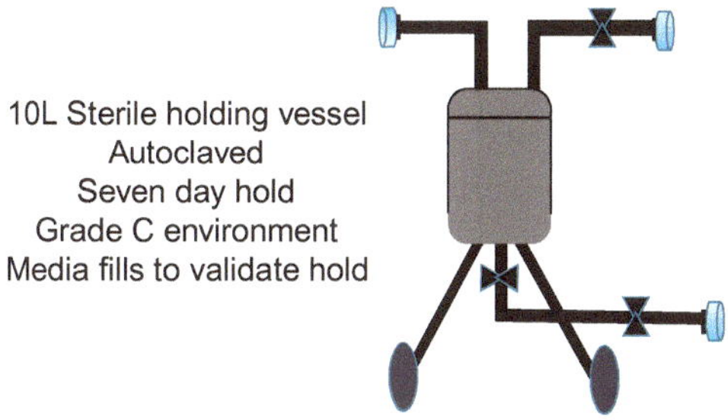

Fig. 4.6 Holding vessel.

the failure during the requalification aseptic process simulation, it did not explain why the initial aseptic process simulations passed. A further investigation of the failure was conducted to uncover a key variable and resulting weakness in the aseptic process.

The initial successful aseptic process simulations took place during a period when there was very low activity was occurring, except for validation. Normal manufacturing had not started yet. The Grade C environment was exhibiting environmental microbial loads closer to Grade A or B environments. During the initial aseptic process simulations, the Grade C area in which the vessel was held was also much cleaner than it would be during normal operations. When normal production began, activities were occurring in the Grade C area and the environment exhibited normal levels of activity and microbial loading. The control system to protect the interior of the vessel from contamination was adequate for the cleaner premanufacturing Grade C environment, but not for the more routine Grade C environment.

The validation study assumed that the Grade C environment was a constant if it met Grade C specifications, but the Grade C environment was a variable. This case study illustrates two important points. First, a careful analysis and evaluation of process variables and the risk they may pose on product quality are needed when designing the process and the validation study. The second point is that aseptic process simulations were not sensitive enough to pick up these weaknesses.

If a properly performed risk assessment was performed, it would likely have identified the wrapped opening on the vessel as potential process weak points as the vessel cooled and the wrapping became wet in the Grade C area. Those designing the system would then have had an opportunity to mitigate that risk with further process controls, such as closing the valves placing the vessel under positive pressure or storing in a more controlled area.

The validation study should then have focused on ensuring that those control measures were effective and reliable. Using the aseptic process simulation could have been a part of that approach, but to identify unaddressed process variables, rather than as the primary means of process qualification.

4.22 Aseptic process simulation study design

An important question to consider when designing the aseptic process simulation study is whether the objective of the study is to provide confidence of aseptic filling operator performance or confirm the capability of the aseptic manufacturing process. Decisions made during the design, such as duration of the aseptic process simulation, inclusion of interventions, and qualification of operators may change depending on what you are trying to do. Human behavior is complex, subject to variability, and unreliable and is difficult if not impossible to validate. The closer one's intent is to qualifying the process, the more effective the aseptic process simulation as a validation tool will be. The closer the intent is to qualifying the person, the more problematic and ineffective it will be.

Whatever the design intent is, a written plan subject to quality review should be in place. This plan should present:

1. intent and objective of the study,
2. clear instructions, written to avoid the potential for individual interpretation, for preference of the study,
3. risk-based rationale for study design, configuration, conditions, and parameters,
4. objective, quantifiable, and measurable acceptance criteria, and
5. provisions for aborting, invalidating, investigating, and addressing deviations related to the study.

A risk assessment should be performed to uncover information needed to make informed decisions on aspects of study design, such as number of runs, number of units to be filled, including worst-case configuration, fill duration, and intervention inclusion.

4.23 When should aseptic process simulations be performed?

There should be written procedures and risk-based criteria or rationales for the frequency of aseptic process simulation studies. Typically, aseptic process simulation studies should be performed for any new or changed aseptic process. The intent of the study is to confirm that the process or process change achieves its intended outcome and that there are no unintended consequences or residual risks introduced by the process or process change that pose a risk or can adversely affect product quality.

Aseptic process simulations should also be performed periodically to determine that unintended or missed changes or variables have not been incorporated into the process that poses a risk to product quality. Aseptic processes are complex, and it would not be realistic to expect that all changes can be captured all the time. To this point, many health authorities have expressed expectations that these periodic studies be performed on a semi-annual basis.

4.24 What process steps should be included in the aseptic process simulation?

As presented in Fig. 4.7, any process steps that may pose a risk or adversely affect the sterility of the product should be included in the aseptic process simulation, unless those steps are adequately validated by some other means or study.

Aseptic process simulations should include such process steps as:

- aseptic additions during compounding,
- product transfer,
- material transfer,
- component transfer,
- fill line setup,
- aseptic connections—including those to sterilizing filter outlets,
- special assemblies—such as PUPSIT (pre-use, post-sterilization integrity test) assemblies,
- inherent (routine) and representative corrective (nonroutine) interventions,
- filling and sealing operations,
- environmental monitoring,
- fill checks conducted in the aseptic processing area,
- shift changes,
- component loading,
- intervention response sanitization,
- lyophilized product transfer and cycle mechanical operations.

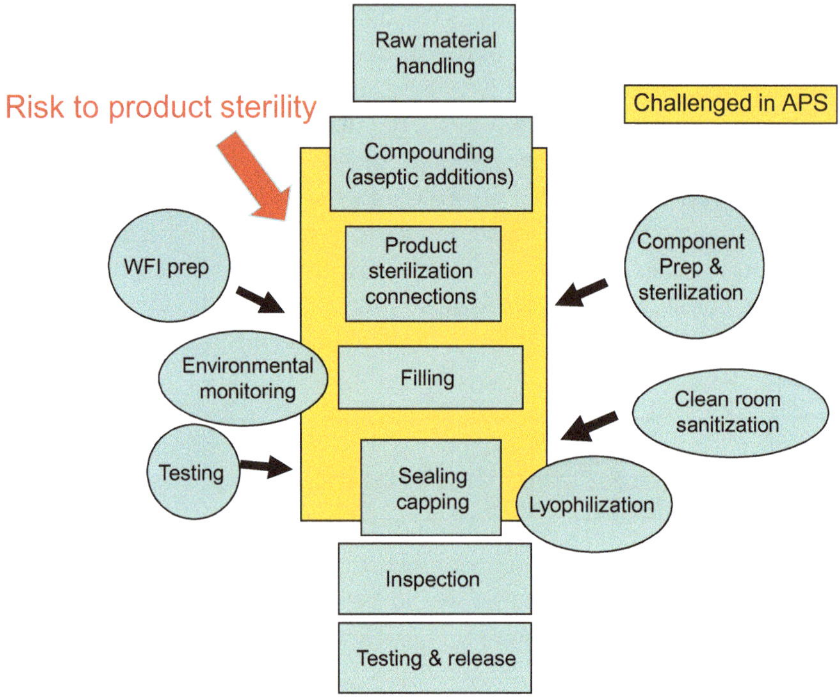

Fig. 4.7 Aseptic process simulation flow chart.

4.25 How many aseptic process simulations should be run for the simulation study?

There should be written procedures and a risk-based criteria or rationale for the number of runs incorporated in the aseptic processing study. Multiple aseptic process simulations should be run for new and modified or changed processes. Typically, three aseptic process simulations are an acceptable number for multiple run studies. Where changes have occurred to processes, multiple runs are prudent to determine the impact of the changes, including unintended consequences of the change and residual risk introduced by the change.

Where there is no evidence of change to the process, as might be the case with periodic aseptic process simulation studies, one run could be sufficient.

4.26 How should the "worst-case" parameters or conditions be included in the study?

The aseptic process simulation should use the configurations, conditions, and aspects of the process that would have the greatest chance of identifying process variability or weakness. This is commonly referred to as "worst-case" conditions.

The rationale for the selection of worst-case conditions for the ascetic process summation should be documented in the validation protocol or document that would be subject to quality review. Worst case in the context of aseptic process simulations does not necessarily mean the worst possible case. It refers to the process parameters and conditions that are most likely to uncover weakness or variability in the process. The worst-case conditions should be used in the process simulation studies to gain the greatest scientific understanding of the process. It can be surmised that if these conditions are challenged in the aseptic process simulations, then conditions representing less than worst case should represent a conservative condition.

In theory, using worst-case conditions is an effective and efficient method to design aseptic process simulations. Unfortunately, defining the actual worst-case parameters and conditions may not always be simple. For example, would the worst case be the maximum or minimum number of operators in the clean room? On the one hand, the maximum number of operators represents the larger source of microbial bioburden, while on the other, the minimum number of operators may mean that operator movement is increased, and their focus on aseptic behavior decreased. Both may represent worst case for different reasons.

Another example would be container size which might be the worst case—the largest container or smallest container. The largest container would have the larger opening, affording more opportunity for contamination to enter, while the small container may be less stable during the transport and filling process. Again, it might not be clear which represents worst case. A final example would be slowest vs fastest fill speed. Slower fills represent longer fill times and a greater opportunity for contamination prior to sealing, however, faster fills may represent more mechanical movement, larger airflow disruption, human activity, and unstable container transport. Without sound justification to identify the worst case from two or more sets of parameters or conditions, then all the potential worst-case configurations should be included in the process simulations study.

4.27 How long should the aseptic process simulation be?

The duration of the aseptic process simulation should be long enough to capture all activities, interventions, and actions relevant to the maintenance of aseptic process performance and product sterility. This will enable it properly to challenge the process to discover any flaws, weakness, or under-addressed variables into the process that can pose a risk to process performance and product sterility. The aseptic process simulations should be long enough to fill sufficient units to capture the low-frequency contamination events that may be present in the aseptic process. Aseptic process simulations should be long enough to properly challenge the process the duration of the aseptic process simulation will also depend on the length of commercial production runs and should capture operator shift changes.

Although a full duration (or longer) aseptic process simulations may be of value in some cases, a risk evaluation may demonstrate that full or longer duration aseptic process simulations are not necessary. In these cases, longer duration aseptic process simulations may lead to a false sense of security and resources could be used more effectively to identify the process risks.

In other cases, longer duration aseptic process simulations may be effective to probe duration-related process variables and conditions that cannot be easily evaluated by any other means. The determination of the duration should be based on scientific, risk-based, and logical evaluation of the objective of the study. The aseptic process simulation should not be used as proof of the acceptability of poor process practices or conditions.

Understanding the objective of the study will aid in determining the duration. For example, if the question is "what is the value of running a full duration aseptic process simulation?" One answer is that the full duration is required to determine the maximum length of time the production run. By digging deeper, it may be possible to understand how the duration of the aseptic process simulation meet provides confidence that the process will be reliable.

Two variables that one may try to address with a long duration fill are (1) whether the environment remains suitable for aseptic processing during the entire length of the fill and (2) whether human fatigue becomes an issue.

Clean room environmental deterioration: The concern is that the clean room environment may deteriorate over the course of the fill and may no longer be suitable for the aseptic process. Since the aseptic process simulation is a secondary output relying on the probability of increased bioburden making its way into the fill, and the fill being properly incubated to detect microbial growth, it is not an effective way to determine or uncover this condition. A much more effective direct measure would be monitoring of the clean room, process, and HVAC system, along with environmental monitoring of viable and total particulate. Since the aseptic process simulation output is a low probability event, is not sensitive enough to determine if the clean room environment has changed sufficiently enough to pose an unacceptable risk to product quality. The aseptic process simulation is not designed to monitor or judge the condition of the environment. The environmental monitoring program will likely indicate that a properly designed and operated clean room environment will remain in control over time. If the clean room environment does deteriorate over time, then the proper response is to provide engineering solutions to address the deterioration and is not to attempt to show that deterioration is still acceptable.

The effect of human fatigue: Clean room personnel can get tired and fatigued. However, aseptic process simulations are ineffective at monitoring human fatigue or the effect of fatigue during aseptic processing because of the difficulty simulating human fatigue. Performing aseptic process simulations for extended periods of time does not probe all the variables associated with fatigue, and each of these may or may not result in a microbial growth. Simply working for extended periods does not consider how much rest or sleep the operation had the night before, or the presence of any nonwork-related stress. The fact that the importance of the test is evident, it also does not probe changes in behavior because the operators are aware that they are participating in a highly observed test.

The best way to address the process variable of human fatigue is by reducing the risk or potential effect human fatigue may have on the outcome of the process. In other words, address the issue by eliminating the cause(s) of work fatigue through better ergonomics, process design, increased rest breaks, and rotations. Running and passing an aseptic process simulation is not the solution for human fatigue.

Note that if operator fatigue is thought to be an important process variable that is mitigated by taking rest breaks, then the aseptic process simulation should include rest breaks. The duration of the aseptic process simulation should include the time the operator enters the clean room between break periods and should include the changes of operators during those break times.

It should also be noted that many global health authorities and regulatory agencies, including the US FDA and EMA, have minimum recommendations and expectations for the number of units filled based on the quantity of commercial batches anticipated. The time it takes to process and fill these units should be considered in planning the duration of the aseptic process simulation runs [3, 5].

4.28 What are the aseptic process simulation acceptance criteria?

The objective of an aseptic process is to produce a sterile product with the absence of microbiological contamination. It follows that the acceptance criteria of the aseptic process simulation should be zero positives.

Any growth should be investigated. The goal of the investigation is to identify the root cause or probable cause of the sources of the contamination. This investigation should include microbiological identification in the positive units and compare them with potential areas where that organism might be found, environmental monitoring results both historical as well as during the fill.

Each possible contamination source should be evaluated to determine if controls and evidence would eliminate that source from aseptic process simulation contamination. Those possible sources that cannot be eliminated should be considered as though they are the source of aseptic process simulation contamination.

CAPAs (corrective actions and preventive actions) should be taken to eliminate each of the remaining causes. After the actions are completed, aseptic process simulation studies should be repeated to confirm both the effectiveness of the CAPAs and that the changes did not have any unintended consequences. Although in general, the number of aseptic process simulation runs may be risk-based, three additional aseptic processing runs should be the default number in response to a CAPA [4, 7].

4.29 The future of aseptic processing

The most innovative new therapies will likely be heat sensitive sterile biopharmaceutical products. It is likely that more of those biopharmaceuticals will be delivered using innovative container and system designs. Therefore, many of the more innovative products will be combination products requiring aseptically processing to manufacture. The cost and availability of these therapies will require and depend on the efficiency, effectiveness, and control of the manufacturing process. The use of advanced technology to achieve the requirements of these products will be essential.

Despite advances in technology in other industries, aseptic processing of sterile medicinal products has struggled to keep up. The reason for this lack of innovation is ultimately due to "keeping the status quo" philosophy because of the perceived risk due to regulatory, change notification, and additional work and time required to support the change.

However, conditions in this industry may be changing and this may be the right time for a technology revolution. This is based in part on the following points:

- Regulators are ready: Global health authorities and regulators are encouraging new approaches. An example is the recent release of the

EMA proposed revisions to Annex 1 (Manufacture of Sterile Medicinal Products), prepared by an international PIC/S working group that included representatives from Europe, United States, Australia, and Japan. The 2107 draft revision contains numerous specific recommendations for risk approaches, with many more implied. This signals the openness by the regulatory bodies for the industry to propose new approaches.

- Manufacturers are recognizing that traditional approaches may no longer fit what we need: The future will involve new and more complex delivery systems as well as sterile ATMP (Advanced Therapy Medicinal Products), Cell and Gene Therapy products, and personalized medicine. These new therapies require aseptic processing. Traditional aseptic processing approaches do not adequately address the unique needs of the manufacturing of autologous sterile products on a very small scale. New (and improved) science and risk-based approaches are needed. The tight release criteria and the timeline for these products will provide an opportunity for rapid microbiological testing, and in-process and real-time release of sterile products.
- Better technology is here and waiting: There is a significant opportunity to acquire and link data at unprecedented levels. This information and knowledge can be used to better model, predict, and control aseptic processes. Simulations along with virtual and augmented reality can be used to significantly reduce costs and timelines for building facilities and developing the process by minimizing change requests and proactively addressing design problems prior to the build-out. Augmented reality can provide more frequent and effective training and expedite qualifications with higher levels of worker skill level and awareness. Artificial intelligence and machine learning can utilize data to optimize processes and process control minimizing variability and improving quality.

  It is important to note that the utilization of technology improvements will require extensive use of automation and knowledge management. As processes become more automated and continuous, process validation will shift from a matter of process testing and replicate runs to qualification of the automated control systems that control process parameters. As manufacturing intelligence and shared data acquisition and utilization systems are used more, the notion of computer system validation based on the US FDA Part 11 and computer software guidance may need to change. Methodologies that have been developed for the software industry [19, 20] may need to be adopted.
- The technology workforce is changing: It is more difficult to attract, train, and retain technical resources. The shortage of skilled, qualified

manufacturing personnel will require industry to rely more on automation and continuous process manufacturing as well as less complex plants. The push toward ATMP will require smaller specialized plants. This aligns well with shifts in the workforce where young high-tech talent is being attracted to the area.

- The return on investment is favorable: Many of the most successful blockbuster health-care products are sterile injectable or implantable produced by aseptic processing. This is a strong business and financial driver for improving the productivity and efficiency of aseptic processes.
- It is the right thing to do: The effectiveness of biopharmaceutical therapies, the demand for these products in emerging growth markets, the cost of health care, and health-care product shortages all emphasize the need for product availability and affordability. In addition to this, shareholder pressure to achieve better returns and performance will drive the industry to seek the best in class manufacturing process efficiency and productivity. This will create a win-win situation for both industry as well as the patient.

The future of aseptic processing lies in the use of technology to meet and exceed the requirements of existing products and new therapies. The time is right to integrate and implement available advanced technologies and further develop new technology. Aseptic processing would benefit from the use of automation, virtual and augmented reality, artificial intelligence, machine learning, and predictive modeling. Technological advances in contamination control using barrier systems, such as isolators and closed RABS, closed container filling, post-aseptic lethal treatments, lower temperature terminal sterilization, rapid microbiological monitoring and testing, methods can significantly reduce the amount of human interaction. Higher productivity and reduced risk can be achieved through continuous process manufacturing, and parametric or real-time release for sterile products. Facilities of the future could be modular with a trend to smaller, less complex, and easier to control critical product exposure spaces. The further development and use of new technology to achieve the required level of aseptic processing improvement can and will result from a partnership of product manufacturers, technology suppliers, and regulators.

4.30 Conclusion: Quality risk management and risk-based critical thinking

The aseptic processing of sterile combination products follows the same requirements and points to consider as the aseptic processing of drug products. The objective of the aseptic process is to *prevent* microbiological contamination of the sterile product and components. This differs from finished product sterilization or terminal sterilization, where the objective is to *eliminate* the microbiological contamination in the product. The prevention of contamination is best achieved through a science and risk-based evaluation of the product and process. This evaluation and analysis should be designed to identify and understand the potential sources of contamination. Understanding the product needs allows for thoughtful design of the process. Understanding the variation and limitations of the process allows for the design of effective control strategies to address variation and minimize process weakness, thus reducing process risk. The use of risk-based thinking has long been encouraged by global Health Authorities. The US FDA mentions it in its 2004 white paper on GMPs for the 21st century and the EU suggests it as a means for process control extensively in its 2017 proposed revision to Annex 1 [4, 18].

Quality risk management involves the use of science and risk-based decision-making. These are methods of critical thinking that help identify risk, causes of risk, and means to reduce risk [21]. The best way to achieve aseptic process control and prevent contamination is to fully understand the capabilities, limitations, and variables of the aseptic process. Product testing, process monitoring, and aseptic process simulations have a role in assuring process control and product quality. Their capability to do so is limited by the process complexity, inherent variation, and lack of established correlations between the observed and actual performance of the aseptic process. Assurance of effective process control can only be truly achieved through risk and science-based aseptic process design practices.

Five simple rules can help meet this objective:

1. *Understand the effects of process steps on other quality attributes of the product.* Identify the contamination-related quality attributes or requirements for the product. Know if the product must be sterile, low bioburden, or endotoxin-free. Map the process steps to determine what impact each step has on the establishment of aseptic process or the prevention of microbiological contamination.
2. *Recognize that failures are the result of unforeseen or under-addressed process variables.* Understand the capability, limitation, and variability of the process steps designed to control, measure, and prevent contamination. While risk is defined as the severity of a hazard times the probability of occurrence times the likelihood of detection of a failure, the best means to reduce risk remains the reduction of the probability of occurrence. Understanding the variability of the process will allow for the implementation of more effective process controls.

3. *Develop and use the best methods available and feasible to control process variability.* Design and choose contamination control strategies and actions that best match the contamination control objective. Do not merely try to monitor or validate risk out of a process. Instead, design controls and technology into the process that reduce risk and address process weakness and variability. Traditional methods of process control that might have appeared to be adequate in the past may not be the best methods available for modern aseptic process controls. Challenge the status quo and strive to innovate. Use the data and information obtained from risk assessments to help drive process improvement.
4. *Be cautious of the unintended consequences on process control measures.* Actions may have both intended and unintended consequences. There may be residual, new, or additional risk, as a result of the unintended consequence of that change.
5. *Understand the metrics for success.* Know the relationship between what can be tested and monitored and the desired or the undesired outcome. Be prepared to interpret and act on the data obtained from monitoring and testing to improve the process. Analysis of trends, even where those results do not exceed limits, may provide valuable predictive contamination control information. Use technology and new approaches where they are available. Even the best processes can be improved.

Exciting new innovations in the biotechnology and personalize medicine areas are challenging the "status quo" of aseptic processing to the limits. Industry and regulators need to embrace technology to enable patients to benefit from these advances. The convergence between high tech (advances in modeling, simulations, and data management), biotech (genetic engineering) with changes in the regulatory environment has created a tremendous opportunity to create new treatment options while minimizing sterility risk to the patient using aseptic practices.

References

[1] US FDA: Guidance for Industry and FDA Staff: Current Good Manufacturing Practice Requirements for Combination Products, January 2017.
[2] US FDA: Title 21: Food and Drugs PART 3—PRODUCT JURISDICTION Subpart A—Assignment of Agency Component for Review of Premarket Applications.
[3] US FDA: Guidance for Industry: Sterile Drug Products Produced by Aseptic Processing—Current Good Manufacturing Practice, September 2004.
[4] EMA, EudraLex, the rules governing medicinal products in the European Union, in: EU guidelines to good manufacturing practice, medicinal products for human and veterinary use, vol. 4, November 2008. Annex 1.

[5] Parenteral Drug Association, Technical Report No. 22, Process Simulation for Aseptically Filled Products, 2011.
[6] Parenteral Drug Association, Technical Report No. 44, Quality Risk Management for Aseptic Processes, 2008.
[7] Parenteral Drug Association Aseptic Processing Points to Consider Part 1, January 2015 and part 2, in: March, 2016.
[8] PDA Presentation by J. Agalloco, Based on the Myth called sterility, Akers, Agalloco, Pharmaceutical Technology, Vol. 34, No. 3, Supplement, Nov. 2010, pp. S 44–45.
[9] Evaluation and Improvement of Aseptic Processes, Risk and aseptic process improvement, baseman, Hanff, long, aseptic and Sterie {processing, control, compliance, and future trends}, Sandell and Tidswell, in: PDA, DHL Publishing LLC, 2017.
[10] US FDA: Guidance for industry an review staff: Target product profile-a strategic development process tool. Target product profile—A strategic development process tool, CDER, Draft, March 2007.
[11] Parenteral Drug Association Technical Report No. 60, Process Validation: A Lifecycle Approach, 2013.
[12] Parenteral Drug Association Technical Report No. 54–5, Quality Risk Management for the Design, Qualification, and Operation of.
[13] International Standard ISO 14644-1 Cleanrooms and Associated Controlled Environments—Part 1: Classification of Air Cleanliness by Particle Concentration, second edition, 2015-12-15.
[14] International Standard ISO 14644-2 Cleanrooms and Associated Controlled Environments—Part 2: Monitoring to Provide Evidence of Cleanroom Performance Related to Air Cleanliness by Particle Concentration, second edition, 2015-12-15.
[15] Parenteral Drug Association Technical Report No. 13, Fundamentals of an Environmental Program, 2014.
[16] US FDA, Guidance or Industry Process Validation: General Principles and Practices Process Validation Guidance, January 2011.
[17] EMA, EudraLex, in: EU Guidelines for Good Manufacturing Practice for Medicinal Products for Human and Veterinary Use, vol. 4, 2015. Annex 15: Qualification and Validation.
[18] US FDA: Pharmaceutical CGMPS for the 21st Century—A Risk-Based Approach, September 2004.
[19] US FDA: Guidance for Industry Part 11, Electronic Records; Electronic Signatures—Scope and Application, August 2003 Pharmaceutical CGMPs.
[20] US FDA: General Principles of Software Validation; Final Guidance for Industry and FDA Staff, January 11, 2002.
[21] EMA: Quality Risk Management (ICH Q9), 31 January 2011, EMA/INS/GMP/79766/2011.

CHAPTER 5

Package/container closures

Thierry Wagner[a], Jennifer Van Mullekom[b], Jane Severin[c], Michael H. Scholla[d]
[a]Dupont, Luxembourg
[b]Virginia Tech, Blacksburg, VA, United States
[c]Network Partners, Warsaw, IN, United States
[d]Dupont, Wilmington, DE, United States

Contents

Assurance of Sterility for Sensitive Combination Products and Materials
https://doi.org/10.1016/B978-0-12-805082-8.00005-0

5.1 History of sterile packaging

The purpose of packaging a sterile health-care product is to allow for sterilization of the product, minimize the risk of ingress of microorganisms, maintain integrity of the sterile barrier system (SBS) overtime and thru environmental and transportation challenges, and allow for aseptic presentation of the product at the point of use. ISO 11607-1 [1, 2] defines the "sterile barrier system" (SBS) as the minimum package that minimizes the risk of ingress of microorganisms and allows aseptic presentation of the sterile contents at the point of use. One of the first examples of an SBS would be Pasteur's swan-neck flask used during the studies he conducted in the 19th century to disprove the theory of spontaneous generation. Pasteur boiled meat broth that would support microbial growth in a flask where the flask had been shaped into a gentle "s." The curve of the glass allowed air into the flask but collected dust and other particles in the bend of the neck. These flasks remained uncontaminated with microorganisms until the neck was removed allowing particles in the air to enter the flask and growth to occur. This experiment also demonstrated the concept of a "tortuous path" which is still utilized today in sterile packaging.

The history of sterile packaging follows the history of medicine and the use of sterile medical instruments during surgery. In the 19th century, the medical practices began the progression into modern medicine because of the increasing knowledge of microbiology proven in the surgical setting by Joseph Lister. Initially, all sterile devices were sterilized at the point of use using carbolic acid and heat. The packaging was metal or glass containers if any at all. Lister could prepare his dressing saturated with carbolic acid within his facility but few other hospitals could copy this technique [3]. Fred Kilmer published his classic article, "Modern Surgical Dressings" in the American Journal of Pharmacy in January 1897 [4] in which he describes the first "commercial" production of sterile surgical dressings. Ultimately, Kilmer joined Johnson & Johnson and true commercial production of sterile medical dressings was started. These were packaged in glass jars and maintained integrity to the point of use wherever they had been shipped.

Packaging of sterile devices also follows the evolution of sterilization methods. In the 1940s, Drs Charles A Phillips and Saul Kaye were assigned to work on biological decontamination at the military base of Fort Detrick [3]. Their work on ethylene oxide (EO) was the basis for commercial use of EO as a sterilant. This opened the doors for device design to incorporate heat labile materials into their construction. EO and radiation sterilization (gamma and electron beam) allowed for the production of single-use disposable medical devices. During the period, medical paper and film packaging became prevalent ultimately joined by DuPont Tyvek[a] in 1972.

In 1976, the United States passed the Medical Device Amendments regulating medical devices [5]. Companies producing single-use sterile medical devices had their own rationales and methodologies for ensuring the packaging maintained sterility to the point of use. During the next 10 years, there was little consensus on this topic and standardized test methods were not widespread. The first attempt to build consensus was in 1993 with HIMA's (now AdvaMed) "Reference on Sterile Packaging" by Curt Larsen, John Spitzley, and Bernie Liebler [6]. The group initiated discussions in the United States on sterile packaging within the industry. At about the same time, the European Union (EU) published its medical device directives and CEN Technical Committee TC102/WG4 developed the EN 868 series of standards for medical packaging and materials. ISO Technical Committee TC198/WG7 was formed and began development of ISO 11607 for packaging of terminally sterilized medical devices. This was closely followed by the US FDA publication of the Quality System Regulation which emphasized validation of product, process, and test methods [7].

The early days of developing the ISO standards for packaging were difficult because of the positioning occurring between members representing CEN interests and those representing the interests of non-CEN member countries. Standards and standards development were new to the packaging industry, and concerns focused on how such standards would be applied. Europe needed a standard that met the essential requirements of the medical device directives, while ISO needed one that was voluntary and applicable globally. The strategy within CEN was to develop a horizontal standard (EN 868-1 [8]) along with several vertical standards to address specific performance requirements for various types of products used in medical packaging (EN 868 Parts 2–10 [9–16]). Conversely, the ISO strategy was to develop a single standard that addressed the required performance attributes of medical packaging without establishing specific performance criteria.

At the meeting of ISO Technical Committee (TC) 198 in Ottawa, ON, Canada in 1993, a resolution was passed with the following instruction: ISO would develop its standard (ISO 11607) and the CEN should develop its standards (EN 868 series) independently. When these standards are

[a]Tyvek is a registered trademarks of E.I. du Pont de Nemours and Company.

revised, efforts should be made to harmonize the ISO and CEN documents. CEN affirmed this approach by passing a resolution with the same strategy. Both committees finished their respective standards, EN 868-1 [8] and ISO 11607, and were published in 1997 [17].

ISO TC198/WG7 began revising ISO 11607 immediately, with a goal of identifying the differences between EN868-1 and ISO 11607. This was a mechanism to show both working groups, ISO TC198/WG7 and CEN TC102/WG4, that the two documents were in fact similar. The results of this work were published as a revised ISO 11607 in 2003. Work began to finally harmonize ISO 11607 and EN 868-1 even before the 2003 revision was published. This effort resulted in the publication of EN ISO 11607-1 and EN ISO 11607-2 in 2006. EN 868-1 was withdrawn and a truly harmonized global standard for medical packaging was created.

During this same time of ISO and EN standards development, and in concert with the initiatives of the Flexible Packaging Association, ASTM committee F2.0 began developing standardized test methods for evaluating medical packaging resulting in the development of over 10 new test methods.

During the next revision of ISO 11607, ISO TC198/WG7 focused on integrating the new requirements of the Medical Device Regulation (MDR) [18] in Europe which made specific references to packaging of sterile medical devices. To maintain compliance with the MDR, the ISO TC198/WG7 working group has incorporated these requirements into ISO 11607 which has been published in February 2019.

5.2 Technologies

5.2.1 Introduction

Combination products bring new challenges for the design and development of packaging systems. A combination product involves a medical device and/or a pharmaceutical and/or a biologic.

The different types of combination products may require different packaging solutions. Packaging needs to keep pace with the rapidly evolving technologies driven to develop innovative products that improves patient outcomes. This product evolution along with changes to sterilization techniques and regulatory pathways are challenging current packaging materials, designs, and processes. These challenges require the packaging professional to be knowledgeable across a wide range of, terminology, materials, designs, processing techniques, sterilization modalities, and regulatory requirements [19–21].

5.2.2 Packaging functions

The function of all packaging systems is to:

1. Protect the product from the environment during sterilization processing, transport, and storage,
2. Communicate about contents and how to safely use the product, and
3. Interface with user to facilitate usage.

The protection of the product from the environmental assaults is a key function of packaging. This includes physical/chemical protection from elements such as mechanical shock, vibration, electrostatic discharge, compression, temperature, light, humidity, and atmospheric pressure changes. Secondary packaging such as corrugated containers provides additional protection during distribution and handling. Tertiary packaging is used for bulk handling, warehouse storage, and transport shipping. The most common form is a palletized unit load [22]. Packages and labels also communicate how to use, transport, recycle, or dispose of the package or product. Packages often have features that interface with the user during distribution, handling, stacking, display, sale, opening, re-closing, use, dispensing, reuse, and recycling. The packaging is typically the first interaction the user has with the product [23–26].

A critical design feature of medical packaging is to enable the user to successfully deliver the product to the sterile field aseptically while minimizing the risk of infection to the patient. For overall risk management, it is important to formally include and evaluate also other usability features like label readability, product identification, etc., in addition to the opening feature, during the design process of a medical packaging system (refer to "Clinical use: aseptic technique and usability aspects").

5.2.3 Differences between requirements of medical device and pharmaceutical packaging

The objective for SBSs for medical device products and pharmaceutical packaging is to ensure that the product remains safe and efficacious. The pharmaceutical and medical device industries have arrived at this solution independently, therefore, it's not surprising that their approach to achieve the same goal is different. Medical devices utilize the ISO 11607 series of documents while pharmaceuticals are guided by the various pharmacopeias.

The medical device standard, ISO 11607-1 for medical packaging, delineates requirements into four areas:

- qualification of materials for safety and performance;
- assessment for sterilization compatibility (see Table 5.1 for material compatibility with various sterilization methods);

Table 5.1 Highlights material compatibility with various sterilization methods [27].

Materials with gas and steam permeability	Permeability sufficient for steam and gaseous sterilisation methods	STEAM at least a part of the packaging needs to be permeable to steam	EO/FORM at least a part of the packaging needs to be permeable to gas	Hydrogen Peroxide (Plasma) natural fibre based materials are incompatible	Gamma/E-Beam or Beta radiation impermeable material may be used	Dry Heat (max temp) impermeable material may be used
Medical grade paper	√	√	√	No	√	√ (160°C)
Flush spunbond non-woven materials of polyethylene	√	√ (max.T 127°C) not suitable for hospitals	√	√	√	no
Wet laid non-wovens (pulp and plastic fibres)	√	√	√	No	√	No
SMS (Spunbond Meltblown Spunbond) non-woven materials of polypropylene	√	√	√	√	No	No
Films and composite films	STEAM at least a part of the packaging needs to be permeable to steam	EO/FORM at least a part of the packaging needs to be permeable to gas	Hydrogen Peroxide (Plasma) natural fibre based materials are incompatible	Gamma/E-Beam or Beta radiation impermeable material may be used	Dry Heat (max temp) impermeable material may be used	

Laminated films, widely used for the manufacture of prefabricated sterile barrier systems (pouches, reels), impermeable						
PET/PP films (PET/Polypropylene)	√	√	√	No	No	
PET/PE films (PET/Polyethylene)	No	√	√	√	No	
Film components, blister materials, high barrier composites, impermeable						
Aluminium laminates and composites, i.e. high barrier materials	√	√	See suppliers specification	√	√	
APET film (Amorphous Polyethylene Terephthlate)	No	√	See suppliers specification	√	No	
E/P (Ethylene-Propylene Copolymer)	see suppliers specification	√	See suppliers specification	see suppliers specification	see suppliers specification	
HDPE film (High Density Polyethylene)	√ (121°C)	√	See suppliers specification	√	No	
LDPE film Low Density Polyethylene	No	√	√	√	No	
PA film (component) (Polyamide)	√	√	√	√	√	

Continued

Table 5.1 Highlights material compatibility with various sterilization methods [27]—Cont'd

Materials with gas and steam permeability	Permeability sufficient for steam and gaseous sterilisation methods	STEAM at least a part of the packaging needs to be permeable to steam	EO/FORM at least a part of the packaging needs to be permeable to gas	Hydrogen Peroxide (Plasma) natural fibre based materials are incompatible	Gamma/E-Beam or Beta radiation impermeable material may be used	Dry Heat (max temp) impermeable material may be used
PE film (component) (Polyethylene)	No	√	√	√	No	
PP film (component) (Polypropylene)	√	√	√	No	No	
PET film (component) (Polyethylene Teraphthalete)	√	√	√	√	√	
PETG (PETG-Foam, PETG-PE) film (PET Glycol)	No	√	See suppliers specification	√	No	
PS film (Polystyrene)	No	√	See suppliers specification	√	No	
HIPS film (High Impact Polystyrene)	No	√	See suppliers specification	√	No	
PC film (Polycarbonate)	√	√	See suppliers specification	√	√	
PVC film (Poly Vinyl Chloride)	No	√	See suppliers specification	No	No	
TPU film (Thermoplastic Polyurethane)	No	√	See suppliers specification	√	√	

- stability testing; accelerated and real-time aging; stable through point of use; and
- physical protection; performance and dynamics testing; shock, compression, puncture, and vibration;
    - o package strength testing; seal strength, material characteristics, and
    - o package integrity testing; no breach of sterile barrier.

Alternately, the pharmaceutical/biologics industry has seemingly more requirements for packaging because the number of products, dosage forms, dosing regimens, packaging components, packaging designs, and materials is immense (Table 5.2).

Table 5.2 An example of the necessary information for a container/closure system to be included in an original drug product application.

Description	Overall general description of the container closure system, plus: *For Each Packaging Component*: • Name, product code, manufacturer, physical description • Materials of construction (for each: name, manufacturer, product code) • Description of any additional treatments or preparations
Suitability	*Protection*: (By each component and/or the container closure system, as appropriate) • Light exposure • Reactive gases (e.g., oxygen) • Moisture permeation • Solvent loss or leakage • Microbial contamination (sterility/container integrity, increased bioburden, microbial limits) • Filth • Other *Safety*: (for each material of construction, as appropriate) • Chemical composition of all plastics, elastomers, adhesives, etc.[1] • Extractables as appropriate for the material[b] Extraction/toxicological evaluation studies, as appropriate Appropriate USP testing Appropriate reference to the indirect food additive regulations (21 CFR 174-186) • Other studies as appropriate *Compatibility*: (for each component and/or the packaging system, as appropriate) • Component/dosage form interaction. USP methods are typically accepted • May also be addressed in post-approval stability studies *Performance*: (for the assembled packaging system) • Functionality and/or drug delivery, as appropriate

Continued

Table 5.2 An example of the necessary information for a container/closure system to be included in an original drug product application—cont'd

Quality control	*For Each Packaging Component Received by the Applicant:* • Applicant's tests and acceptance criteria • Dimensional (drawing) and performance criteria • Method to monitor consistency in composition, as appropriate *For Each Packaging Component Provided by the Supplier:* • Manufacturer's acceptance criteria for release, as appropriate • Brief description of the manufacturing process
Stability	• See section III.C.4

FDA 'Guidance for Industry Container Closure Systems for Packaging Human Drugs and Biologics' page 22, May 1999 [24].

5.2.4 Container types/definitions/dosage form

There are numerous container types and dosage forms, including packaging systems and features that are not necessarily terminally sterilized, but are hermetic or tightly closed. As dosage forms evolve, future systems may offer a solution for a novel product that also requires terminal sterilization.

The United States Pharmacopeia (USP) classifies containers by their ability to protect their contents from the external environment. At a minimum, the container must be *well closed to* protect the contents from contamination under ordinary conditions of handling, storage, and distribution. A *tight container* protects the contents from contamination by extraneous liquids, solids, or vapors, from loss of the article, and from efflorescence, deliquescence, or evaporation under the ordinary or customary conditions of handling, storage, and distribution, and is capable of tight reclosure. A *hermetic container* is impervious to air or any other gas under the typical conditions of handling, shipment, storage, and distribution. Sterile hermetic containers generally hold preparations intended for injection or parenteral administration. A *light-resistant container* is intended to provide protection from light (Fig. 5.1).

Containers are further categorized based on the number of doses it contains. A *single-dose container* is one that holds a quantity of drug intended as a single dose and when opened cannot be resealed with confidence that sterility has been maintained. These containers include fusion-sealed ampules and prefilled syringes and cartridges (Fig. 5.2).

A *multiple-dose container* is a hermetic container that permits withdrawal of multiple doses from the contents without impacting the strength, quality, or purity of the remaining contents, for example, vials (Fig. 5.3).

Parenteral products are administered by breaching the skin barrier. This common effective method of delivering combination products enables

Fig. 5.1 Container/closure system commonly used for solid dosage forms (tablets or capsules). *iStock.com/CollinsChin*

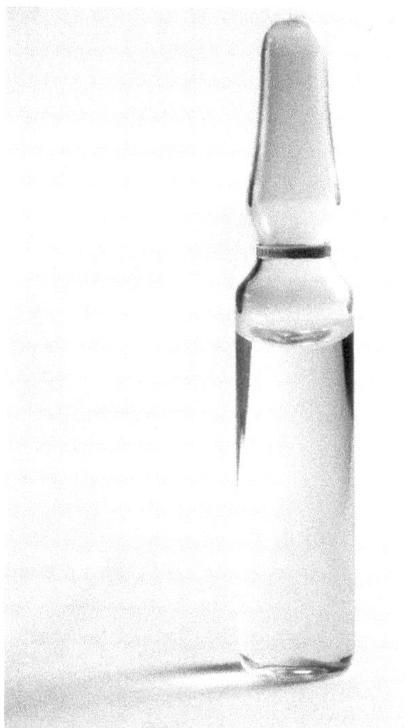

Fig. 5.2 Fusion-sealed ampule—example of a single-dose container. *iStock.com/ambassador806*

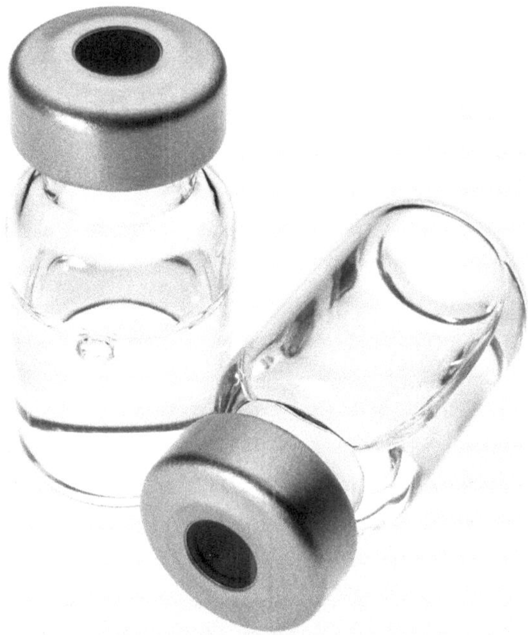

Fig. 5.3 Glass vial—example of a multidose container. *iStock.com/FreezeFrameStudio*

increased bioavailability by bypassing the skin, however, it introduces additional challenges for package development. In addition to maintenance of sterility, parenteral delivery requires controls to minimize particulates, endotoxins, extractables, and leachables. Examples of containers and closures for parenterals include plastic IV bags, prefilled syringes, vials, and ampules. The USP lists five primary types of preparations intended for parenteral administration:

- *Injection*: liquid preparations that are drug substances or drug solutions
- *For injection*: dry solids that upon reconstitution, yield solutions that must meet all requirements for injections
- *Injectable emulsions*: liquid preparations of drug substances dissolved or dispersed in a suitable emulsion
- *Injectable suspension*: liquid preparations of solids suspended in a suitable liquid
- *For Injectable suspension:* dry solids that, upon addition of suitable vehicles, yield preparations conforming in all respects to the requirements of injectable suspensions [28] (Fig. 5.4 and Table 5.3)

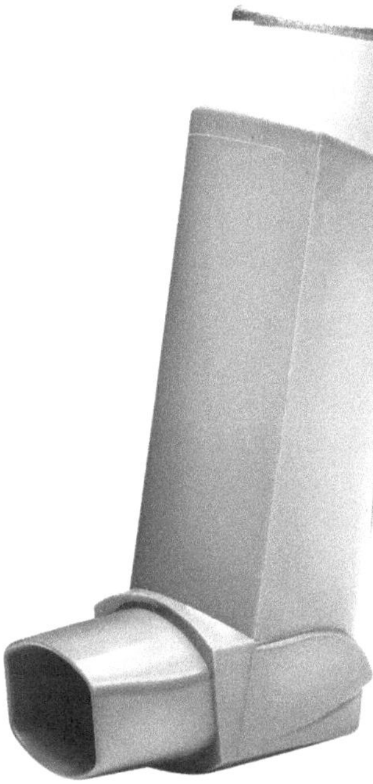

Fig. 5.4 Inhaler device. *iStock.com/csheezio*

Table 5.3 Categories of packaging systems and examples.

Bulk	Unit-dose/non-reclosable	Multi-dose
Bottle (Plastic and Glass)	Pre-filled syringe	Vial
Sacks/Bags	Blister packs	Bottles (Plastic and Glass)
Drums/Kegs	Blow-fill-Seal (BFS)	Tubes
	Ampules	Aerosols
	Vials	Ophthalmic/Otic solution or suspension Delivery Systems
	Injection/Infusion Systems	Metered Dose Inhalers
	Sachets	

5.2.5 Considerations for plastic selection-pharmaceutical and medical device packaging

Table 5.4 illustrates the correlation between the degree of concern regarding the route of administration with the likelihood of packaging component-dosage form interactions for different classes of drug products. To appropriately select plastic materials for a terminally sterilized package,

Table 5.4 Examples of packaging concerns for common classes of drug products.

Degree of concern associated with the route of administration	Likelihood of packaging component-dosage form interaction		
	High	**Medium**	**Low**
Highest	Inhalation aerosols and solutions; injections and injectable suspensions[a]	Sterile powders and powders for injection; inhalation powders	
High	Ophthalmic solutions and suspensions; transdermal ointments and patches; nasal aerosols and sprays		
Low	Topical solutions and suspensions; topical and lingual aerosols; oral solutions and suspensions	Topical powders; oral powders	Oral tablets and oral (hard and soft gelatin) capsules

FDA 'Guidance for Industry-Container Closure Systems for Packaging Human Drugs and Biologics' page 6, 1999 [24] www.fda.gov/downloads/drugs/.../Guidances/ucm070551.pdf.

it is crucial to understand the input parameters and their possible ranges. Examples of parameters include proposed sterilization method, temperature, duration of exposure, pressure, and sterilant composition. Second, a thorough understanding is required of the impact of those inputs on packaging materials, the product contained therein, and any interactions between packaging and product. This includes the possible physical-chemical degradation or changes in material characteristics, properties, and safety, throughout the shelf life of the product post-sterilization. The basic functions of packaging are covered in Sections 5.2.4 and 5.2.5. The specific considerations encountered that should be carefully evaluated when selecting types of plastic are (a) permeability of the containers to atmospheric oxygen and to moisture vapor, (b) leaching of the ingredients of the container structure to the internal contents, (c) compatibility assessment, (d) absorption of drugs from the contents to the container, (e) transmission of light through the container, and (f) storage conditions generating extractables from the container and/or label into the product. Agents frequently added to change the properties of plastic include plasticizers, stabilizers, antioxidants, antistatic agents, antifungal agents, colorants, and others.

Extractables are compounds that can be extracted from packaging materials, such as elastomeric, plastic components, or coating on the container or closure system, when exposed to certain solvents, harsh environmental conditions, or processing. Leachables are compounds that leach from the packaging as a result of direct contact with the formulation of the drug product and then potentially impact the drug or device and possibly passed on to the patient. It is important for the manufacturer to conduct risk assessments when designing products to identify areas of concern. Long-term and accelerated stability studies are performed to assess the safety of the product for the desired shelf life [29].

Liquid pharmaceuticals packaged in permeable plastic may lose drug molecules or solvents through the container altering the concentration of the drug in the product thus affecting its potency, properties, and stability. Sorption is the binding of molecules, which includes both adsorption (takes place on the surface of a substrate) and absorption (a substance enters the 'bulk' of the other material; e.g., the container wall). Sorption occurs through chemical or physical means due to the chemical structure of the solution molecules and the physical and chemical properties of the polymer. The sorption of a pharmacologic agent from a pharmaceutical solution could reduce its concentration and affect strength of the product. The sorption of pharmaceutical excipients such as colorants, preservatives, or stabilizers could also impact the product formulation. The solution pH may influence the sorption tendency of the solution, and the pH of a solution may also affect the chemical nature of a plastic container.

Deformations, softening, hardening, and other physical changes in plastic containers can be caused by the action of the container's contents or external factors including changes in temperature and the physical stresses placed upon the container in handling and shipping [23, 24, 29, 30].

5.2.6 Stability issues related to packaging

Numerous factors can affect the stability of a drug or device including pH, temperature, solvent, light, air (oxygen), carbon dioxide, moisture or humidity, and particle size. The barrier properties of the packaging can have a profound impact on the stability of the product. Permeability of carbon dioxide can impact pH, and the solvent itself may escape the container. Permeability to air (oxygen) can induce degradation via oxidation. Degradation can be minimized by filling the container as much as possible to minimize the headspace, or by filling the headspace with nitrogen. Another option is to add an antioxidant to the formulation. Carbon dioxide can cause insoluble carbonates to form in the solid dosage form, which decreases the disintegration and dissolution properties of the product. Packaging in tight containers and filling the containers as full as possible minimize this condition [22–24]. Degradation of pharmaceuticals as well as label materials can be induced by light. The effects of light can be minimized by packaging products in light-resistant containers; products that are light sensitive can be covered during administration with aluminum foil or an amber plastic overwrap.

5.2.7 Challenges for packaging combination products

As the development of combination products continues to evolve, so will the challenges to effectively and economically package them. New technologies need to address unmet needs result in increasingly complex packages. The packaging industry must keep pace with the rapidly evolving development of new materials, sterilization methods, and technologies to deliver these critical therapies to the patients safely and effectively.

One example of a new challenge is the packaging of biologics. The Center for Biologics Evaluation and Research (CBER) states 'In contrast to most drugs that are chemically synthesized and their structure is known, most biologics tend to be heat sensitive and susceptible to microbial contamination. Therefore, it is necessary to use aseptic principles from initial manufacturing steps which is also in contrast to most conventional drugs' [31]. 'Biologic products often represent the cutting-edge of biomedical research and in time may offer the most effective means to treat a variety of medical illnesses and conditions that currently have no other treatments available.' Biologics are from the human body or other biological entities, such as vaccines, etc. These products are labile and very challenging to package. A typical medical device may be packaged and sterilized and have a shelf life of 5 years, while a biologic may only be shelf stable for weeks. This type of product will likely require a new method of filling or packing and the development of compatible packaging materials. New materials intended to contain biologics will likely require maximum barrier properties as these biologics are sensitive to moisture, temperature, UV light, as well as oxidation. Many combination products provide convenience for the user to deliver a drug dose. Examples include prefilled syringes, insulin injector pens, transdermal patches, metered dose inhalers, etc. In this case, a device can be the drug container, the primary package as well as the delivery device (Fig. 5.5).

It is essential that packaging as well as sterilization are considered very early in the development planning and design control for a device/combination

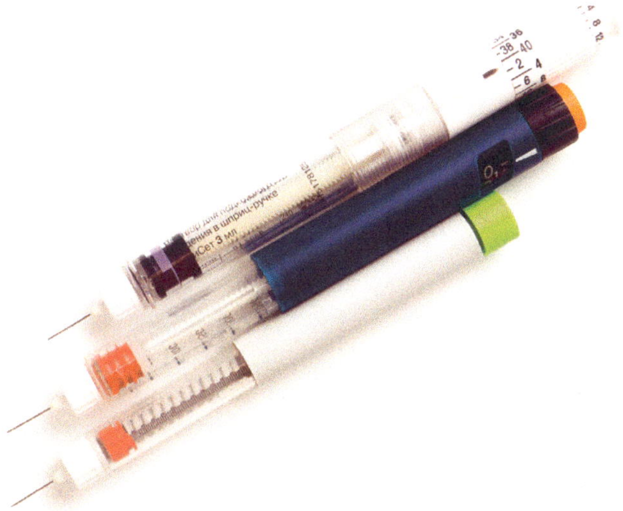

Fig. 5.5 Prefilled injector pens. *iStock.com/Kuruan*

product to avoid expensive changes later in the process. A complete requirements definition must be developed for the development of a packaging system. Careful identification of 'packaging design inputs' such as technical requirements, user needs, and 'packaging design outputs'; acceptance criteria, specifications, and drawings need to be documented. This is followed by packaging design verification where laboratory performance tests are conducted to confirm the design inputs meet the design outputs. Finally, packaging design validation is conducted to provide objective evidence that design meets the user requirements [23, 24, 32–35].

5.3 Validation principles

5.3.1 Validation and patient safety

Health-care-associated infections (HAIs) continue to be one of the highest frequency adverse events in the delivery of health care. Achieving and maintaining sterility of medical devices or combination products with an adequate SBS while at the same time facilitating the aseptic presentation during use are key factors in the fight against HAIs. To this end, the design of a SBS must be carefully planned and validated. The forming, assembly, and sealing or closure processes must be developed reliably through validation. Validation is a crucial activity for establishing, securing, and maintaining sterile conditions since sterility of the device, the medicinal product, or its combination cannot be verified at the point of use. In addition to patient safety requirements, the health-care industry is faced with the need for increased efficiency and productivity in order to drive down costs. Carefully designed validation approaches along with reliable test methods, and process control tools enable leveraging of data that can dramatically reduce the costs of changes and keep them to a minimum.

5.3.2 Package integrity and the limitations of sterility testing

Sterility testing has been used in the past to verify the sterility of products but it only provides a false sense of security since the conclusions that can be drawn from sterility test data have significant limitations. Sterility testing can only detect microorganisms that are viable, but testing is dependent on culture media and growth conditions. Testing for all types of microorganisms and all conditions is impractical. In addition, the sterility tests are destructive, take days to complete and are prone to false positives. This often leads to inconclusive root cause analysis if results are positive for microbial growth. Most importantly, the low incident rates require extremely large sample sizes to generate meaningful conclusions for sterility. For example:

Assume the hypothetical case where sterility testing is used for accepting or rejecting a batch of packaged sterile devices with a sterility assurance level, SAL $=10^{-2}$. In this case, one item out of hundred from this batch would potentially be non-sterile, vs the normal objective of one in a million. With only one tested sample, the probability to accept that batch is $1-10^{-2}$ or 99%. With two tested samples, the probability to accept the batch would be $(1-10^{-2})\times(1-10^{-2})=98\%$. We can deduct the following formula:

Probability to accept a batch with SAL $=10^{-2}$ with n samples tested for sterility: $p=(1-10^{-2})^n$.

Using this formula for 20 samples, the batch is accepted in 82% of the cases, with 50 samples accepted in 50% of the cases and with 300 samples the batch would still be accepted in 5% of the cases. The typical target of a SAL of 10^{-6} would require far more samples. One can easily conclude that with a SAL of 10^{-6}, the equation will be: $p=(1-10^{-6})^n$ and millions of samples will be required to achieve similar confidence. Obviously, the practicalities of manufacturing millions of samples to destructively test them are prohibitive.

5.3.3 Test methods

Test methods are the cornerstone of all validation. An accurate and reliable method to assess the output is required to make informed decisions.

Package testing has focused on seal integrity for both nonporous and porous pouches, to demonstrate that they protect product from microbial ingress. Other key methods are microbial barrier testing of porous materials and seal strength testing.

ISO 11607-1 annex B [36] includes an informative list of test methods and guidance documents that may be used to demonstrate compliance with requirements of ISO 11607-1. ASTM F2097 [37] is another useful guide for test methods selection. A useful detailed guidance is also provided in annex A of ISO TS 16775 [38] on "*Selection, evaluation and testing of packaging materials and sterile barrier systems.*" Fundamental material properties such as tensile strength, elongation, puncture, tear resistance, and abrasion resistance can also be monitored.

5.3.3.1 Integrity test methods

Test methods to assess the integrity of seals and closures are arguably the most important of the test methods used for the validation of SBSs. Seal integrity shall *"minimize the ingress of microorganisms"* into the packaging [1]. For nonporous SBSs, there is an additional requirement to ensure that the gas surrounding the product is also preserved. USP <1207> [39] defines package integrity for nonporous packaging as "*the ability of a sterile product container–closure system to keep product contents in, while keeping detrimental environmental contaminants out.*" Thus, for nonporous sterile containers, integrity is confirmed if a package allows no leakage greater than the maximum allowable leakage limit.

The sensitivity of the test is the probability of detection of a given integrity defect, for example, the critical leak rate or critical hole size. Critical parameters are dependent on the packaging type, product type, defect type, and environmental exposure of the package itself. These factors have been studied and reported in the literature. Morton and Kirsch confirmed that microbial ingress does not occur for leak rates lower than 10^{-5} Pa m^3/s. Kirsch et al. also showed that for gas leak rates of 10^{-4} Pa m^3/s, liquid leakage would not always occur, while the probability for microbial ingress would be even lower. Various articles, like those of Kirsch et al. published in the PDA Journal from 1997 to 2000, or Burrell et al. [40] and Keller et al. [41] concluded that in containers for sterile liquids critical defect sizes as small as 0.3–10 μm may lead to loss of sterility. They further demonstrated that a liquid must be present for microbial ingress to occur. He concluded that liquid leakage and microbial ingress are probabilistic events, while gas leakage is a deterministic event. Since the shape of real defects may differ significantly from perfect round holes and some may represent a tortuous path, the defect leak rate is a more reliable measure compared to the dimension of defects to determine what is critical and what is not. Dana Morton Guazzo provides an excellent summary in Michael J. Akers' book "Sterile Drug Products" [42].

The validation of integrity test methods requires defining the critical defect size that is detectable, followed by demonstrating it can be measured with acceptable repeatability. For packaging of solid articles like medical devices, the main concern is to protect against airborne microbial challenges rather than the ingress of liquids. In the case of a defect or hole of a given size, the leak rate will be a function of the differential pressure between the inside and outside of the package as well as the packaging porosity. The goal of porous packaging is ensuring it remains a microbial barrier while being permeable to gas. This has enabled gaseous sterilization modalities to be used extensively and efficiently on a large variety of products while maintaining sterility. Porous packages are also efficient in reducing differential pressures while air can penetrate through numerous tortuous pathways minimizing the impact of a potential defect. Hacket et al. concluded in a series of experiments in 2000 that "*using a material with high permeability in a well-designed package can provide an effective barrier system even when a hole of 25 μm or smaller is present*" [43].

The most used integrity test method is probably visual inspection based on ASTM F1886 [44]. Extensive round robin data have been documented with channels of 125 μm being detected at 94% and 75 μm detected at 79%. Visual inspection has limitations in terms of sensitivity and reliability if operators have to perform the test over longtime periods. For this reason, it is not always accepted by authorities. Nevertheless, it is an excellent method for routine checks, but cannot replace other more sensitive methods that are required for state-of-the-art validation.

Dye penetration testing for porous packaging as per ASTM F1929 [45] is capable of detecting leaks as small as 50 μm with a probability of 99%. The bubble test (ASTM F2096 [46]) is a popular test and easy to realize. Its main weakness is the lower sensitivity with porous materials. Customized methods have been developed to test porous lidded trays with CO_2 tracer gas (ASTM F2228) or with vacuum decay methods (ASTM F2338 [47]). These nondestructive tests have acceptable sensitivities, but they required customized equipment and are significantly more expensive. Recent developments in ultrasound testing (ASTM F3004 [48]) or optical tomographic imaging are also encouraging since these tests can be used online

Table 5.5 Sensitivities of integrity test methods for porous packaging.

ASTM test	Type of test	Test focus	Destructive?	Hole/channel size
F1886	Visual inspection	Seals	No	75 μm
F1929	Dye penetration	Seals	Yes	50 μm
F2096	Internal pressurization bubble test	Package	Yes	250 μm
F2228	CO_2 tracer gas	Package (porous area masked)	No	50–100 μm
F2338	Vacuum decay	Package (porous area masked)	No	100–125 μm
F3004	Airborne ultrasound	Seals	No	Depending on defect type (750 μm)

on packaging machines, but require further optimization. Table 5.5 provides an overview of sensitivities of commonly used integrity test methods for porous packaging.

5.3.3.2 *Integrity testing—Conclusions*

Numerous publications and studies have concluded that microbial ingress methods are not reliable due to their probabilistic nature. The low frequency and random nature of defects require large sample sizes and sophisticated equipment. For this reason, they are not practical to validate and implement. On the other hand, deterministic methods that are based on physical phenomenon, predictable, and easily controlled (USP <1207> [39]) are recommended and preferred. Nonporous packaging relies on leak testing as well as dye ingress testing. Porous packaging often uses the dye ingress tests which remain popular and well accepted. Despite their destructive nature and messiness, dye ingress tests are capable of detecting defects with acceptable sensitivity, low cost, and easy to implement and validate.

5.3.3.3 *Microbial barrier test methods*

Harmonization of medical packaging standards between ISO and CEN started in the 1990. One area of focus was microbial barrier test methods because the available standards were not globally recognized. After years of experimentation with whole package tests and failure to consistently validate those tests, scientists and regulators concluded that integrity testing of seals and closures and separate microbial barrier testing of porous materials is significantly more reliable [49, 50].

Tallentire and Sinclair developed a fundamental understanding of the penetration of particulates in narrow channels. By correlating particulates and spores, they concluded, that microbial barrier performance can be predicted when testing with particles instead of spores [51, 52]. This created the basis for the development of ASTM F2638 [53]. Herman and Larsen gave an excellent overview on these developments [54]. After the method was recognized by the FDA in 2013 [55], DuPont used it extensively for equivalence testing comparing data of "transition" Tyvek produced on the newer manufacturing lines and" legacy" Tyvek produced on the older manufacturing lines within the framework of the medical packaging transition project. The method is accepted by many authorities such as Health Canada, notified bodies in Europe, CFDA in China, and others.

Research in whole package testing is still active, despite the issues described above to validate these methods (see Dunkelberg et al. [56–58] or Severin et al. [59]). Current research explores the challenges of microbial ingress testing from aerosolization. The goal of this research is to arrive at a barrier method that allows the user to control the other variables such as pressure, humidity, and temperature. This ability allows the user to design experiments to qualify their packaging systems under 'real-life' conditions. The main challenge to this research is the variation of the input variables such as specific organisms, as well as process variables such as microbial growth and recovery. While variability is an issue, the inability to detect critical size holes continues to be the main issue for validation. With new technologies, research will probably continue, however, these methods will likely remain fundamental research tools rather than useful tests for packaging validation purposes.

5.3.3.4 Seal strength test methods

Seal strength is a critical quality attribute for the validation and control of sealing processes. Meeting a defined mechanical strength of seals can be important for compatibility with sterilization processes, and is certainly important for a package being able to withstand the stresses of transport and handling. Two test methods are mainly used in the industry, ASTM F88 [60] and according to the annex D in EN 868-5 [61] which will also refer to ASTM F88 in its new version (Fig. 5.6 and Table 5.6).

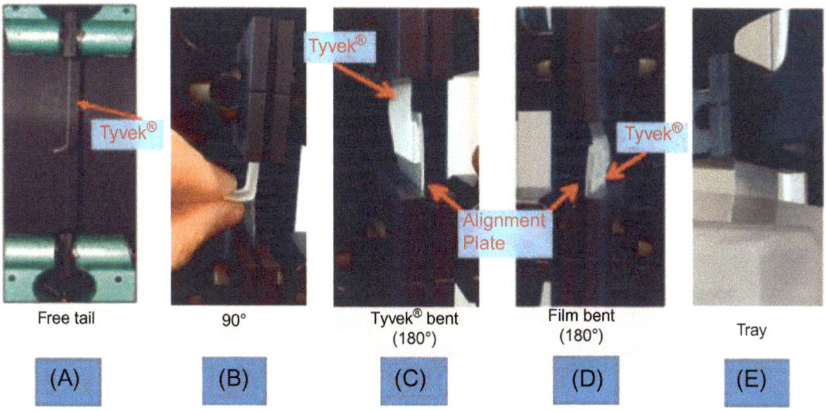

Fig. 5.6 Seal strength measurement techniques.

Table 5.6 Seal strength measurement techniques details.

Technique	Tail holding
A	Unsupported ("Free Tail", angle can vary throughout the test)
B	Supported 90° (Fixed Angle by hand or better using a support)
C	Top Web Bent (supported 180°)
D	Film/Bottom Web (supported 180°)
E	Free Tail Lid Material Upper Bent 180°

The strategic development of validation protocols enables industry to assure safety to the patient while implementing efficient and cost-effective packaging systems. A model example of this is when Dupont made a global change in Tyvek raw material. Tyvek has been used extensively for packaging undergoing gaseous-based sterilization modalities because of its unique permeability and long successful history. DuPont provided a path that enabled their customers to transition smoothly from the older legacy Tyvek to a new product by working closely with global regulatory bodies as well as their customers. This enabled the Tyvek transition without individual medical device companies revalidating all their products which would have resulted in product disruptions to the patients and higher cost without improving safety of the products.

In 2015, DuPont published the results of the equivalence testing protocol comparing "transition" Tyvek® produced on the newer manufacturing lines and "legacy" Tyvek® produced on the older manufacturing lines. This included over 50,000 seal strength measurements, 78 different packaging applications marketed by 55 medical device manufacturers throughout the world. DuPont supported their customers by gaining alignment with the regulatory bodies which included providing data with multiple methodologies to support the change assessments and notifications.

5.3.3.5 Validation of test methods

Validation of packaging test methods has been a subject of intense discussion in the medical device industry since the introduction of ISO 11607 "*Packaging for terminally sterilized medical devices*" in 2006. Unlike the medical device industry, the pharmaceutical industry has diligently embraced the concept of validation in analytical procedures for identification, and quantification of impurities and active ingredients. US and European pharmaceutical products regulatory requirements are captured as a part of good manufacturing practice (GMP) (US: 21CFR211.165, EU:Volume 4 EU Guidelines to Good Manufacturing Practice [62], guidance in ICH Q2(R1) [63] accepted by the FDA, EU, and Japan). The purpose of validation is to provide documented evidence to demonstrate that a method fulfills the requirements for its intended use, in other words, that it is suitable for its intended use.

The ASTM made significant contributions in the area of test method validation with its rigorous approach for conducting interlaboratory studies to determine the precision and bias of a test method (see ASTM E691 [64]) The precision is determined by establishing the repeatability or the variability between measurements produced by the same equipment and operator, respectively, the reproducibility or the variability between measurements between different test equipment, operators, and/or test laboratories. The precision and bias section, included in each standard, gives an indication about the limits of detection of the method as well as the typical variability, which is required when selecting adequate test methods and when implementing the test method in a laboratory.

Test method selection, implementation, validation can be onerous tasks and it is important to keep the identified risk to the patient in mind in relation to packaging design aspects to be assessed. Validation should cover limits for the intended application and not the method's theoretical capability. Guidance for SBS test method validation can be found in annex O of ISO TS 16775 [38]. General principles and definitions are available in ISO 5725-1 [65], a basic method for the determination of repeatability and reproducibility is proposed in ISO 5725-2 [66].

5.3.4 Design validation

Design validation and process validation of a specified SBS are two distinct activities, although they are done together. Design validation includes performance and stability testing. Aspects related to SBS sterility need to be validated, however, there are elements of the design that can be verified by checking that design outputs meet design inputs. Key elements include the qualification of materials including aspects of biocompatibility, package dimensions, position of the device in the packaging, and the presence of the label as specified.

5.3.4.1 Material qualifications, chemical, and biological compatibility

ISO 11607-1:2006—Section 5.5 addresses the physical, chemical, environmental, and biological requirements of materials used in the manufacture of SBSs. Many of these requirements are guaranteed by suppliers of preformed SBSs. Manufacturers may have to assess certain specific properties themselves for material qualification during the qualification of their suppliers or for routine incoming quality control to satisfy quality management system, respectively, regulatory requirements.

5.3.4.2 Microbial barrier properties

Porous materials used for SBSs allow the sterilization gases to enter and exit the package while preventing the ingress of microorganisms based on a defined porosity. ISO 11607-1 requires that microbial barrier properties are evaluated to be adequate, without further indication about what "adequate" means. As a horizontal standard, ISO 11607 "*Packaging for terminally sterilized medical devices*" applies to a wide range of different sterile barrier solutions, which could be small or very large, and which could be used in very different environments and conditions over shelf lives ranging from months to decades. This evaluation will be dependent on the specific application, the targeted environment, the analysis of risks, and the specific regulatory requirements. The new upcoming European MDR [67] requires risks to be "acceptable" and "*compatible with a high level of protection of health and safety, taking into account the generally acknowledged state of the art.*" It requires also to eliminate or to reduce as far as possible the risk of infection to patients and to design to "*prevent microbial contamination of the device or its content such as specimens or fluids.*"

5.3.4.3 Biological compatibility and toxicological attributes

It is a regulatory requirement to demonstrate the compatibility between the sterilized device and the impacted biological tissues of the patient. This includes the impact of the packaging in contact with the device. Plasticizers, additives, impurities, residues of polymer catalysts, endotoxins, adhesives, inks, and particulates that transfer can impact the safety of the device or pharmaceutical. Depending on the type of product and risks, the assessment may range from a description of the composition of the packaging material and an evaluation of cytotoxicity to a detailed risk analysis with targeted testing depending on the type of patient contact and its duration. ISO 10993-1 *Evaluation and testing within a risk management process* [68] provides a framework for biological evaluations. The ISO 10993 series of documents provides guidance on appropriate testing to address specific identified risks. ASTM F2475 *Standard Guide for Biocompatibility Evaluation of Medical Device Packaging Materials* [69] helps with specific aspects of packaging materials. The evaluation of biocompatibility can be a complex undertaking and it is recommended to research specialized literature [70] and consult experts.

5.3.4.4 Extractables and leachables

The degree of rigor needed in determining the potential interactions between packaging and the drug product is a function of the dosage form and the route of administration as well as stability testing requirements. The FDA Guidance for Industry on *Container Closure Systems for Packaging Human Drugs and Biologics* [24] includes three degrees of concern in function of the dosage form (Table 5.2). The EU Guideline on *Plastic Immediate Packaging Materials* [71] describes the requirements for marketing authorization applications to be submitted for packaging materials in direct contact with the active substance or medicinal product. The guideline includes a decision tree based on the dosage form defining the type studies and documentation required. Nonsolid active pharmaceutical ingredients (API) require the complete qualitative composition of the plastic material if pharmacopeia compliance of the immediate packaging material cannot be demonstrated. Many leachables are detected during initial material qualification studies, however, some negative interactions might only appear during stability studies. Toxicological data are required for extractables and leachables. Selecting materials with a known chemical characterization can significantly shorten the development process. Selecting materials that are compliant with food contact regulations or with compendial pharmacopeia monographs can reduce the regulatory burden significantly.

5.3.4.5 Performance qualification

The objective of performance testing is to demonstrate maintenance of integrity of the SBS by testing the entire packaging system, which includes the SBS packaged and its protective packaging, after handling, distribution, and storage and after exposure to expected condition (ISO 11607-1:2016: paragraph 6.3 [72]). Demonstration of preservation of product performance is typically done at the same time.

Defining the distribution and storage environment

According to the ISO 13485:2016 paragraph 4.2.3 [35], the organization has to include "*specifications or procedures for packaging, storage, handling and distribution*" into the medical device file. Products must be protected from alteration, contamination, or damage when exposed to expected conditions and hazards. ASTM D4169 [73] and ISTA guidelines [74] provide the basis for testing packaging systems to demonstrate that they are suitable for the intended use. Testing should be done with the device or at least a surrogate with similar weight and shape. Establishing worst-case scenarios enables leveraging data over packaging and device families.

Clinical use: Aseptic technique and usability aspects

In addition to the packaging being a barrier, the packaging must facilitate the aseptic presentation of the medical device during use in the clinical environment. In ISO 11139 [75], aseptic presentation is defined as "transfer of sterile contents from its sterile barrier system using conditions and procedures that minimize the risk of microbial contamination." Observations in health-care facilities highlight the differences in the level of training and approaches to managing sterile fields and handling packages. The increased attention to the causes of HAIs has resulted in increased awareness on aseptic presentation. Trier et al. [76] documented a very interesting study in 2014 showing that contamination rates can indeed be significant. Regulations include requirements for medical device designs (including their SBSs) to enable easy and safe handling to minimize the risks of infections, and consequently manufacturers need to include aseptic presentation in their formal risk analysis. This topic needs to be considered in the broader context of usability of the device with its SBSs, which also covers aspects such as labeling and the ability to assess SBS integrity. ISO 11607-1 [72] currently does not provide specific design recommendations to facilitate aseptic presentation. The revised version of ISO 11607 likely to be published end of 2018 will include a new requirement to conduct a "*usability evaluation for aseptic presentation*" with a focus on a few key aspects that provide some insights into necessary design features. The Sterile Barrier Association has published a guidance document on aspects to consider for usability of SBSs, which includes aseptic presentation [77].

5.3.4.6 Stability studies

The classification of a combination product's primary mode of action defines the regulatory pathway. In Europe, the first case will be regulated under the medical device or active implantable medical device directives [78, 79], the second case will be under the directive for medicinal products [80]. This is particularly important for defining the procedures to follow for stability testing as regulations will not be cumulative. Stability studies tend to take considerable time and are resource intensive, so it is important to seek advice and support.

ISO 11607-1 "*Packaging for terminally sterilized medical devices*" Part 1 [1] requires stability studies of the SBS based on real-time aging to demonstrate the maintenance of integrity overtime, however, accelerated aging results are considered sufficient to go to market when real-time aging results are not yet available. The standard also requires real-time and accelerated aging tests to begin simultaneously. This ensures that both sample populations are comparable, facilitating root cause analysis in the event that there are unexpected results. Accelerated aging duration is typically calculated based on ASTM F1980 [81] with elevated temperatures while normally staying below 56 °C or lower. The Arrhenius equation is used to correlate real-time aging and accelerated aging as a function of temperature. The rate of chemical reactions doubles with every temperature increase of 10 °C, up to approximately 60 °C. This correlation often decreases at greater temperatures increasing the risk of failures [81]. For this reason, it is good practice to proceed conservatively to avoid repeating these time consuming and expensive studies.

Stability studies for the packaging itself can be leveraged if the same packaging is applied to different devices and when it is demonstrated that "*the product does not interact with the specified sterile barrier system over time*" (ISO 11607-1 paragraph 6.4.7) [36].

For drug products, the requirements for stability testing for products marketed in the United States are defined in CFR §211.166 [82]:

> *(a) There shall be a written testing program designed to assess the stability characteristics of drug products. The results of such stability testing shall be used in determining appropriate storage conditions and expiration dates. …*

The European Directive 2001/83/EC [80] requires submission of a description and the specifications of the container and the closure system(s) for the active substance(s) and a summary of the detail of the stability studies, including "*information on the analytical procedures used to generate the data and validation of these procedures.*" It requires also to provide a "*post-authorization stability protocol.*"

Under 3.2.2.2. "*Pharmaceutical development*" directive 2001/83/EC states.

(g) The suitability of the container and closure system used for the storage, shipping and use of the finished product shall be documented. A possible interaction between medicinal product and container may need to be considered.

The International Council for Harmonization of Technical Requirements for Pharmaceuticals for Human Use (ICH) issued a series stability study guidelines. These documents have been adopted by the United States, Europe and Japan, and other regulatory agencies. The documents can be downloaded on the ICH website under quality guidelines [83] and are also available through the FDA in the United States, EMA in Europe, and PMDA in Japan.

SBSs and product stability studies are typically conducted together. When the drug or device stability is explored concurrently with packaging, interactions will also be captured (see FDA guidance: Early Development Considerations for Innovative Combination Products [32]). As per ICH Q1A (R2) [84] Guideline for "*Stability Testing of New Drug Substances and Products*" "*The stability studies should be conducted on the drug substance packaged in a container closure system that is the same as or simulates the packaging proposed for storage and distribution.*"

5.3.5 Forming, sealing (closure) and assembly process validation

Validation of processes is a key quality management system requirement (ISO 13845 [35]) when *"the resulting output cannot be verified by subsequent monitoring or measurement.* "A number of guidance documents referred to by the Center for Devices and Radiological Health (CDRH) of the United States Food and Drug Administration (US FDA) and other national authorities for medical devices help define the process: the Global Harmonization Task Force (GHTF) document GHTF/SG3/N99-10:2004 [85] or *Guidance for Industry Process Validation* by the US FDA [86]. The US FDA guidance applies a life cycle approach to process validation linking processes development, qualification, and routine monitoring to ensure the process is maintained in a state of control. The GHTF document [85] includes a list of elements to be included for the development of a validation protocol and provides a detailed annex on statistical methods and tools to help designing capability/studies, control plans, designed experiments, gauge R&R studies and data analysis as well as approaches for determining sample sizes. It also advocates for a risk based and a quality-by-design approach. It defines process validation as "*the collection and evaluation of data, from the process design stage through commercial production, which establishes scientific evidence that a process is capable of consistently delivering quality product.*" A key to this approach is to understand the drivers of product variation and take the appropriate control based on risk. ISO 11607-2 "*Packaging for terminally sterilized medical devices*" part 2 defines the validation requirements for forming, sealing, and assembly processes for SBSs [2]. It also addresses the various packaging system life cycles including process control and monitoring. Further guidance is available in ISO/TS 16775: packaging for terminally sterilized medical devices—Guidance on the application of ISO 11607-1 and ISO 11607-2 [38].

5.3.5.1 Process design

Annex A of ISO 11607-2 "*Packaging for terminally sterilized medical devices*" part 2 [2] provides guidance on process development. ISO 11607-2 [2] requires the definition of critical process parameters, their set points, and tolerances to produce packaging that meets the establish specifications. The FDA guidance [86] takes a different approach by evaluating parameters commensurate with their risk to the process and the process output, regarding "*criticality as a continuum rather than a binary state.*" In that sense, the 2019 version of ISO 11607-2 will require the establishment of a process specification and will discontinue the concept of critical process parameters.

ISO TS 16775 [3] proposes a structured process for the packaging design including process development. Annex Q provides guidance on establishing process parameters and Annex S provides guidance on process design evaluation. This is aligned with a quality-by-design approach for pharmaceutical and medical products which focuses the effort at the front-end of the project instead of inspecting quality into the product.

5.3.5.2 Installation, operational, and performance qualifications

The Global Harmonization Task Force (GHTF) guidance [85], the US FDA guidance [86], and ISO 11607-2 propose slightly different definitions to the concepts of installation qualification (IQ), operational qualification (OQ), and performance qualification (PQ). A major initiative has started in 2013 within the ISO TCs for sterilization to harmonize definitions throughout the suite of sterilization, aseptic processing, and packaging standards [75].

ISO 11607-2 defines IQ and OQ as the process of obtaining and documenting evidence that equipment adheres to its specification and operates within predetermined limits when used in accordance with its operational procedures. The language of the definitions has slightly changed in the 2018 version based on ISO 11139 [75]. The PQ demonstrates that the process "*under anticipated conditions, consistently produces a product ... which meets all predetermined requirements*" considering all sources of variability. The US FDA guidance includes the concepts of IQ and OQ into "equipment qualification" and defines the process performance qualification (PPQ) as the step to "*confirm the process design and demonstrate that the commercial manufacturing process performs as expected.*" The Global Harmonization Task Force (GHTF) guidance and ISO 11607-2 include under OQ to run the process based on the established parameters resulting from process development to assure that the process output actually meets the defined requirements under all anticipated conditions of manufacturing. The objective of the PQ is to assess the long-term capability while considering sources of potential variability such as machine start-ups, different operators or shifts, material lot-to-lot differences, change over procedures.

5.3.5.3 Process control and monitoring (continuous process verification)

Process development should also specify the process variables and attributes and acceptance criteria for continuous monitoring or scheduled testing. Under the FDA, these measures are defined as "*continuous process verification.*" All these measures along with the acceptance criteria should be included during the PQ.

The validation activities require substantial testing and deviations and/or failures may be observed during the various process validation exercises. The expectation is that the validation should include root cause investigation as well as any corrective or preventive actions.

5.3.6 Packaging and device families

Validation is an essential activity, but it can be an extensive undertaking. Significant leveraging of cost and time can be achieved if the validation is performed for entire packaging or medical device families.

ISO 11607-1 [72] includes a key statement that is the basis for establishing packaging families:

> *"6.1.6 When similar devices use the same packaging system, a rationale for establishing similarities and identifying the worst-case configuration shall be documented. As a minimum, the worst-case configuration shall be used to determine compliance with this part of ISO 11607.*
> *NOTE For example, similarity could be established by different sizes of the same product."*

ISO 11607-2:2006/Amd:2014 [2] includes a similar statement in paragraph 5.1.5. It further states under 5.1.4, that validation may rely on data from previous IQ and OQ. If a machine is used for several SBSs, it is good practice to perform a machine focused IQ and OQ to set the basis for a reliable and properly validated equipment. Care should be taken to ensure that the machine IQ/OQ limits cover the extremes of all the SBS sealing process windows. It is recommended that product-specific OQ and PQ elements are covered in a separate study. This is also important in case of changes to or repairs of the packaging machine. In this case, only the machine-specific aspects have to be repeated.

5.3.7 Managing changes and revalidation

Control of design and development changes is a key quality system requirement [7, 35] which obviously also applies to packaging. ISO 13485:2016 [35] further clarified under 7.5.7: "*Processes for sterilization and sterile barrier systems shall be validated prior to implementation and following product or process changes, as appropriate.*" In addition to reviews after changes, periodic reviews should be conducted to detect any changes that went unnoticed or combinations of minor subtle changes that together can compromise the state of validation. The Notified Body Operations Group (NBOG) in Europe issued in 2014 new guidance on *Reporting of Design Changes and Changes of the Quality System* [87], explicitly labeling changes to the packaging process as "substantial." It further states: "*Changes in packaging characteristics of a sterile medical device, configuration or density could affect the absorption or penetration of the sterilant, the residue levels (where applicable) and the effectiveness of the sterilization process in addition to the safety of the sterile device. Issues of compatibility between the packaging material and the sterilization process must also be taken into consideration to ensure that seal integrity is not affected and that the packaging preserves the functionality and safety of the device throughout its declared shelf-life.*"

Wagner and Scholla published an article in 2013 [88] summarizing the regulatory requirements for revalidation of sterile packaging. They recommended a structured risk-based approach for the validation steps that allows the revalidation effort to be limited to those areas that are affected. This can have a significant effect on time and cost. There is a growing expectation by regulators to improve products based on market feedback and documented CAPA. With this background, ISO Technical Committee TC84 has created a new working group (WG 15) in 2014 to address Device Change Management for pharmaceutical products. The committee draft document has been published in 2016 and recommends a risk-based approach to establish a level of verification and to take a "*step-wise approach to testing… until such time that the data is sufficient to support a scientifically valid conclusion that the benefits outweigh the risks.*" The document should be useful to provide guidance and clarity on how partial revalidations can be tailored avoiding unnecessary testing while maintaining a high degree of protection of the patient.

Managing changes and revalidations is an essential part of each products life cycle. As the regulatory scrutiny increases, the impact of design upgrades or unexpected changes can be minimized by careful design of the initial validation paying close attention to some of the issues previously discussed.

5.3.8 Examples of validation approaches

Validation is the process to generate data to provide objective (typically scientific data) evidence that the requirements for a specific intended use or application have been fulfilled. The intended use requirements for the validation of sterile packaging can be summarized with the following key questions:

- Can the worst-case SBS withstand the hazards of distribution, handling, and storage without losing integrity?
- Does the SBS maintain integrity over the entire shelf life?
- Is aseptic presentation possible as planned under all intended circumstances?
- Is the peeling and opening behavior within specifications over the entire shelf life?
- Is the packaging process in statistical control, repeatable and does the packaging meet specifications even under worst-case conditions taking into account all sources of variability?
- And in case of a change, is the new material functionally equivalent to the previously validated material?

Developing the questions to be answered is the key input for developing a good validation protocol. The protocol should clearly identify the objectives of the validation including all information necessary for its execution, data analysis, and final reporting. See Fig. 5.7 for an example of a sterile packaging validation protocol outline.

Fig. 5.8 shows an example of a validation work flow based on the one presented by N. Kaller, Packaging Engineer at DuPont in a webinar in 2014 [89]. Please note that this example is based on the definitions of IQ, OQ, and PQ of ISO 11607-2 [2]. The approach will be slightly different if the US FDA guidance for process validation [86] is used or the Global Harmonization Task Force (GHTF) validation guidance [85].

Example of a sterile packaging validation protocol outline

- Introduction
- Objectives
    - o Design validation, process validation, revalidation … indicate what is covered, indicate key questions to be answered
- Product & process description
    - o Device description and requirements
    - o Packaging specification
    - o Packaging and Product Families
    - o Worst case consideration
    - o Process Workflow
    - o Transportation, distribution and storage environment
- References
- Regulatory requirements
- Test methods
    - o Rational for selection of test methods
    - o Acceptance criteria
    - o Sensitivity for integrity test methods
    - o Test equipment
    - o Validation of test methods
- Validation Resources
    - o Internal team and responsibilities
    - o Third party test labs support
- Study Design
    - o Process validation
        - ▪ IQ
        - ▪ OQ
        - ▪ PQ
        - ▪ Process control measures
    - o Sterilization
    - o Design validation
        - ▪ Stability testing
        - ▪ Performance testing
        - ▪ Clinical evaluation
- Data from previous studies
- Sampling and data handling Procedures
- Statistics
- Documentation and test report requirements
- Quality control and assurance
- Time line
- Attachments

Fig. 5.7 Example of a sterile packaging validation protocol outline.

Fig. 5.9 shows an alternative approach for a validation workflow as proposed by the Sterile Barrier Association [90]. Interesting aspects of this approach is that it includes the creation of a baseline at time zero. This data can be used as a reference to compare to accelerated aging and real-time aging data. This is essential to draw final conclusions and for root cause analysis in case of problems. Another interesting aspect is that product used for accelerated aging and real-time aging has been exposed first to performance testing

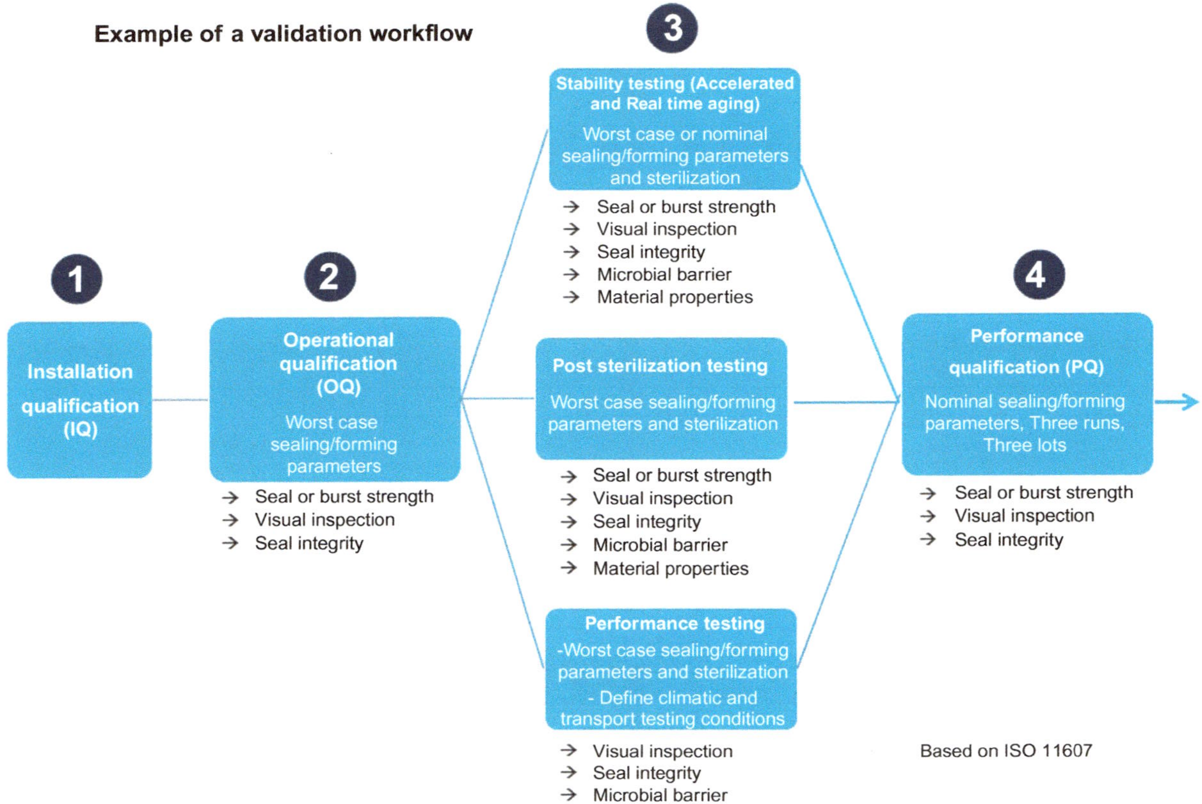

Fig. 5.8 Sample validation flow diagram.

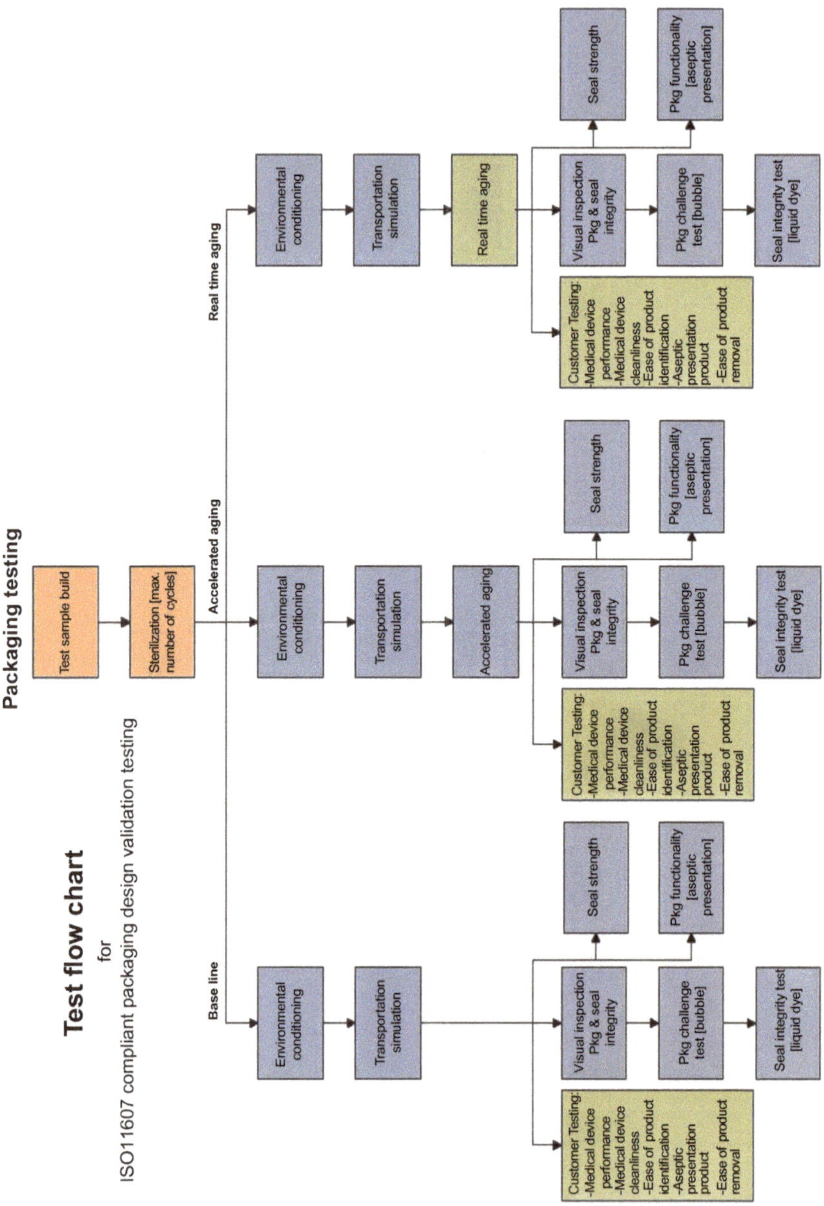

Fig. 5.9 Test flow chart as proposed by the sterile barrier association (www.sterilebarrier.org).

to challenge the packaging through a simulated distribution environment. The approach depends on the device, the packaging, the supply chain to deliver the product, and the risk management approach of the manufacturer. A rationale should be developed as a justification. As discussed earlier, although it is typical to conduct performance and stability testing separately, a validation engineer might decide to conduct performance testing serially after accelerated aging if, for example, the product is shipped to the hospital up to the end of the shelf life from a consigned stock. This would be particularly important if the packaging has decreasing performance at the end of aging.

Fig. 5.8 lists a number of typical tests that are normally performed like seal strength, burst strength, visual inspection, seal integrity (dye penetration), microbial barrier of porous materials, and mechanical properties of the packaging materials. The validation flow in Fig. 5.9 uses the bubble test [46] to assess the integrity of the entire pack. Bubble testing is popular, since it is one of the only tests to assess the entire packaging although its sensitivity of 250 μm is limited.

5.4 Power and sample size considerations for medical and pharmaceutical device packaging

5.4.1 A conceptual overview of power and sample size

Statistical hypothesis testing forms the cornerstone for answering technical questions in the development, quality assurance, and meeting regulatory requirements of medical device and pharmaceutical packaging. Such testing provides the evidence for ensuring patient safety during change management and achieving validation requirements as described in Section 5.3.1. Statistical techniques can be used to analyze data generated to characterize SBSs and package systems as related to their performance. The following list contains examples of the technical questions that may be answered with hypothesis testing:

- Does the packaging maintain its properties after aging?
- Which film provides the highest package integrity?
- Is a suggested component equivalent to an obsolete one?
- Is the packaging process capable?

This section will address power and sample size requirements as related to hypothesis testing and process capability.

The statistical concepts of power and sample size are crucial to ensuring valid hypothesis tests and sound application of the scientific method. Power and sample size will be addressed from a practitioner's view point in this section. In layman's terms, power can be defined simply as the ability to detect an effect if there truly is one. For example, power is a measure of the ability to demonstrate a process change lowered package seal strength if the change truly did lower seal strength. In statistical terms power is P(Rejecting $H_0 | H_1$ is true), where H_0 is the null hypothesis and H_1 is the alternative. Please refer to Moore et al. [91] for a more thorough treatment of hypothesis testing.

A definition of the elements of power and sample size calculations is in Table 5.7.

Typically, an alpha value is set at either 5% or 1% depending on the impact of falsely detecting an effect. The effect size is set from technical expectations or industry benchmarks. Power is typically set at 80% or 90% for the minimum effect size. Sample size is often limited due to the experimental budget in the form of cost and/or time. Care should be taken to obtain an estimate of the standard deviation from a random, representative historical sample.

Table 5.7 Elements of a power calculation.

Element	Description and examples
α (alpha) or Type I Error Rate	• P(Rejecting $H_0 \| H_0$ is true) • α can often be described as the chance of falsely detecting an effect. • There is a 5% chance of falsely detecting the process change reduced seal strength
Δ or Effect size	• The minimum expected change • The new package design should increase yield from 93% to 97%, an effect size of 4%.
Power	• P(Rejecting $H_0 \| H_1$ is true) • Power can be described as the ability to detect an effect if there truly is one. • There is an 80% chance of detecting a 2% increase in dye penetration from the old configuration to the new configuration.
n or Sample size	• The number of items to be tested. • Note that many statistical software packages provide sample size in number per group versus the total sample size. Before implementing a test plan, verify whether the software supplies the total sample size or the sample size per group.
Standard deviation	• A measure of the spread of the data, typically obtained from historical experimentation or process operations.

Table 5.8 The impact of increasing an input to a power analysis with all other quantities fixed.

Increase in input	Power
α (alpha) or Type I error rate	↑
Δ or effect size	↑
n or Sample size	↑
Standard deviation	↓

A conceptual understanding of power and sample size calculations includes an understanding of how the various elements affect calculations relative to one another. Table 5.8 provides a summary of these relationships, assuming all other quantities are fixed. For example, assume the experimenter increases α or the type I error rate keeping all other quantities fixed. This change will increase the power for a given effect size, sample size, and standard deviation. If the experimenter increases the assumed effect size for the study, keeping all other quantities fixed, then the power for the experiment increases. Note the opposite of the impacts in Table 5.8 holds when the quantities listed in the first column decrease. Power is a complex nonlinear relationship, specific to the hypothesis being tested. One should always investigate the impact of a range of plausible values for power analysis inputs for the specific case of interest.

5.4.2 A power and sample size example for packaging

A power and sample size analysis that explores multiple options is most useful in developing an experimental strategy. Assume that a packaging engineer wishes to evaluate a new film that promises an increase in seal strength of 0.6 lb/in at the current processing conditions and compare it to the current or control film. The historical standard deviation for the process is 0.2 lb/in. Alpha is set at 0.05 and an acceptable value for power is determined to be 80%. To be conservative, the engineer decides to explore scenarios of a minimum effect size from 0.2 lb/in to a maximum of 0.6 lb/in.

Multiple statistical software packages perform power and sample size analysis. JMP® and Minitab® are two popular graphical user interface (GUI) packages among statistical practitioners in science and engineering. SAS and R offer code-based options with R being an open source package, free to download. Fig. 5.10 shows the result of a two sample *t*-test power analysis from Minitab® statistical software under the alternative hypothesis that the mean of the test film is greater than the mean of the control film. Note the sample size quantities in Fig. 5.10 are per group.

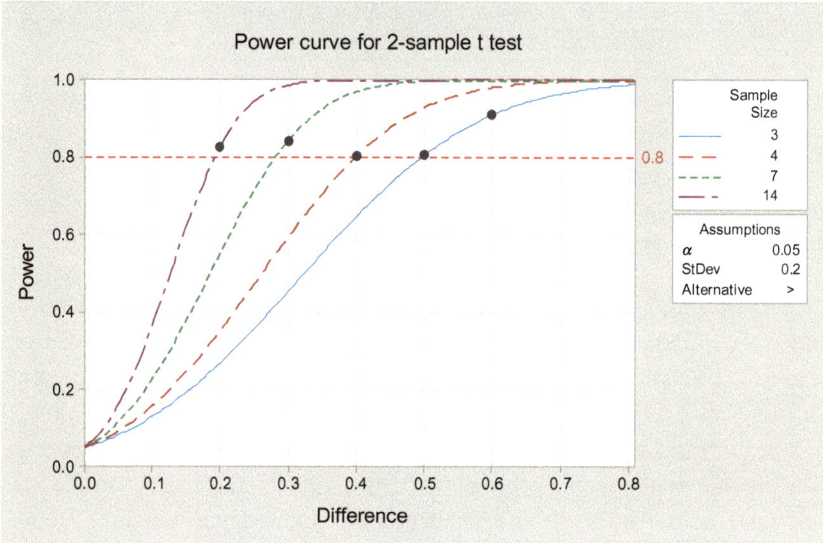

Fig. 5.10 Power Curve Example.

Table 5.9 Summary of power and sample size analysis from Fig. 5.10.

Effect size	Sample size (per group)	Total sample size (control + test)
0.2	14	28
0.3	7	14
0.4	4	8
0.5	3	6
0.6	3	6

The power curves in Fig. 5.10 show that in order to achieve the benchmark power of 80% the sample sizes required per group are as designated in Table 5.9. Smaller effects require larger sample sizes to detect.

For illustrative purposes, the aforementioned example is simplified. Of course, the sample sizes in Fig. 5.10 and Table 5.9 assume that the engineer has selected at random, representative sample using a validated test method with emphasis on measurement system validation. Any special cause variation such as batch-to-batch variability, equipment drift, or bias among tensile force testers could lead to biased conclusions. Best practices in experimentation require that the experimenter either minimizes this variability or design an experiment which accounts for it. It is important to note that minimizing variability through limiting the scope of the experiment may limit the generalizability of the results. Furthermore, in order to avoid selecting a sample size that is too small resulting in an underpowered experiment, the standard deviation estimate used in the power analysis must account for each such source of variability in order to power the experiment to detect affects over and above the extraneous sources. For example, one would not want to use a standard deviation for one operator and one test apparatus to plan the test when multiple operators and multiple tests stands are to be used in the execution of the test. The additional operators and test stands will introduce additional variability and make the test plan based on one operator and one test plan underpowered.

5.4.3 Power and sample calculations in practice for significance testing

Power and sample size calculations are easily performed in a variety of statistical software packages for testing for statistically significant differences. They are too numerous to be detailed in this text. Table 5.10 contains a list of commonly used statistical tests and their applications for continuous variables (i.e., seal strength) while Table 5.11 contains the same information for discrete measures (i.e., defect counts). Care should always be taken to ensure that data meet the assumptions required for statistical tests including normality, independence, or expected count minimums. For additional information on assumptions, see Moore et al. [91].

Table 5.10 Common tests of statistical significance for continuous variables.

Application	Hypothesis test	Example
Determine a mean difference from a target	One sample t	Is the process on aim for seal strength?
Determine a mean difference in two groups	Two sample t	Do the two packaging lines differ in seal strength?
Determine a difference in standard deviation (or variance) among groups	Equal variance tests: Bartletts Levene	Is the variation different among the four packaging lines?
Determine a mean difference in more than two groups	One Way ANOVA	Is the average seal strength different among the four packaging lines?
Determine if there is a linear relationship between two continuous variables	Simple Linear Regression	Can I predict seal strength based on sealing temperature?

Table 5.11 Common tests of statistical significance for discrete variables.

Application	Hypothesis test	Null hypothesis
Determine a difference in percentage or proportion from a target.	One sample proportion test	Is the proportion of packaging defects below 0.1%?
Determine a difference in percentage or proportion in two groups	Two sample proportion test	Do the two proposed configurations differ in their dye penetration rates?
Determine if percentages or proportions are equally distributed among groups	Chi-squared goodness of fit tests	Is the proportion of defects produced equally distributed among the four manufacturing lines?
Determine if the percentage or proportion chance of falling in categories of one variable depends on another	Chi-squared test of Independence	Does the type of defect classification vary based on the film type used?
Determine if there is a relationship between a binary outcome (i.e. pass/fail) and a continuous variable	Binary Logistic Regression	Does the percentage of fiber tear vary based on the seal strength?

Tables 5.10 and 5.11 are intended to aid the experimenter in translating research questions to statistical hypotheses and perform appropriate power and sample size calculations in statistical software. The practitioner is encouraged to consult the software documentation on each of these software packages for the specific details of the inputs and interpretation of the respective power and sample size calculations. A word of caution related to testing a hypothesis that involves groups such as the two sample *t*-test and analysis of variance (ANOVA) is in order. Most software provides you the sample size per group meaning that the user would have to multiply by the number of groups.

The general linear model and multiple linear regression represent extensions of the one-way ANOVA and simple linear regression, respectively, for multiple independent variables that are beyond the scope of this discussion.

5.4.4 An overview of equivalence testing

Statistical significance testing is used to determine if quantities are significantly different than one another. However, experimenters often have a need to determine if quantities are equivalent within some practical margin. Determining equivalence is particularly relevant for change management protocol, ensuring consistent global quality, and qualification of multiple testing laboratories. It is important to note that finding no significant difference does not allow for a conclusion of equivalence. Statistical theory prevents this, allowing only for the conclusion of "there was not enough evidence to indicate a significant difference." As its name implies, equivalence testing can be used to determine the equivalence of quantities within a prespecified bound. See Stein and Doganoksoy (1999) [92] for an overview of equivalence testing. Equivalence testing requires subject matter experts, not statistical practitioners, to determine the appropriate equivalence bounds.

There are many articles in the statistical literature regarding equivalence testing. The approach in this section is based on the original two one-sided test (TOST) approach by Schuirmann (1987) [93]. Equivalence testing for a test vs control group employs the two sample t-test. Differences in significance testing and equivalence testing can be summarized in Table 5.12 and Fig. 5.11.

5.4.5 Power and sample size considerations for equivalence testing

In equivalence testing, the role of consumer's risk and producer's risk is reversed from their typical alignments of types I and II errors, respectively. In addition, equivalence testing power includes the additional input of the region of functional equivalence. The power and sample size depend on the location of the difference relative to 0 (effect size), the location of the

Table 5.12 Summary of statistical significance and functional equivalence.

Analysis	Statistical significance	Functional equivalence
Statistical technique	Student's *t*-test	Student's *t*-test
Confidence level	95%	90%
Interpretation	Demonstrates control and test material are significantly different	Demonstrates control and test material are equivalent within a pre-specified margin

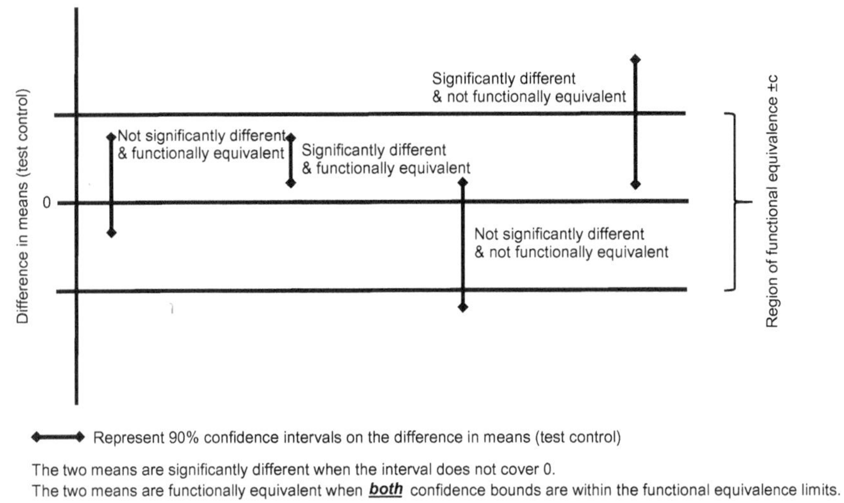

Fig. 5.11 Interpretation of statistical significance and functional equivalence.

difference relative to the equivalence bounds (equivalence limits), and the variability. Several statistical software packages offer power and sample size calculations for equivalence testing.

5.4.6 Sample size for process capability in process validation

Many medical packaging and pharmaceutical manufacturers are concerned about the amount of data required for collection in process stability and process capability during validation. There is no specific formula to provide a sample size for determining process control and capability. However, there are guiding principles and tools that can be used to make decisions in the face of uncertainty.

First, one must have an understanding of the source of variability in the process and ensure that data are taken over a time period that allows observation of these sources. For example, if a manufacturing process is known to vary by raw material batch, then one must ensure production is observed over multiple batches vs just one batch to include this source of variability into the validation effort. If equipment is known to drift over the months, then one day of data from a production line is not sufficient for process validation. A team approach to identifying these sources of variation is best. The team should include all relevant personnel from technical, quality, and operations areas.

Once the sources of variability have been observed over a sufficient time period, a runs chart can be used to check for stability, trends, oscillation, etc.

Runs charts and associated hypothesis tests are available in many software packages for examining the stability of a process.

Many students of statistics have heard of the magic sample size number of $N=30$ and apply it stability and validation cases. One of the reasons for the recommendation of $N=30$ is related to obtaining a precise estimate of the standard deviation for process capability. Nelson [94] created a nomograph that indicates the standard deviation reaches an error percentage of <10% at $N=30$ for standard normal distributions with 95% confidence. In contrast, a sample of $N=10$ could have error as high as 26% in the standard deviation. Biased estimates of standard deviation are particularly problematic in process capability calculations, thus the more data for estimating the standard deviation, the better. Of course, this is assuming all impactful sources of variation have been observed.

An example in the context of C_{pk} is explored to further characterize the sample size required to achieve a particular process capability. Recall

$$C_{pk} = \min\left(\frac{\bar{X} - LSL}{s}, \frac{\bar{X} - USL}{s}\right) \tag{5.1}$$

where $\bar{X}$ is the sample mean, s is the sample standard deviation, and LSL and USL are the lower and upper specification limits, respectively.

While $N=30$ provides a reasonable error percentage for standard deviation, this sample size may not be large enough to indicate that process capability is above a particular threshold. An observed C_{pk} of 1.4 may be above 1.33, however, a $C_{pk}=1.40$ is a point estimate with no reflection of the uncertainty in the estimate. There are two important factors that help a manufacturer determine if C_{pk} is above a prespecified threshold with a particular level of confidence. They are the observed C_{pk} from the sample and the sample size.

A 95% lower confidence interval approach is used to conclude if the process capability is above a threshold, often 1.33. The formula for the confidence interval, denoted by LCL, is given in Eq. (5.2) (Montgomery, 2009) [95].

$$LCL = \hat{C}_{pk}\left[1 - Z_{\alpha}\sqrt{\frac{1}{9n\hat{C}_{pk}^{2}} + \frac{1}{2(n-1)}}\right] \tag{5.2}$$

This bound should be greater than a specified minimum threshold, such as 1.33. The value of $Z_{0.95}$ is 1.64 and n is the sample size. $\hat{C}_{pk}$ is the estimate

Table 5.13 Lower confidence limits for selected sample sizes and sample values of $\hat{C}_{pk}$.

	$\hat{C}_{pk}$ (calculated from the sample)			
Sample size	**1.33**	**1.50**	**1.75**	**2.00**
10	0.79	0.90	1.05	1.20
20	0.96	1.08	1.27	1.45
30	1.03	1.16	1.36	1.56
50	1.10	1.24	1.45	1.66
100	1.17	1.32	1.53	1.76
200	1.21	1.37	1.60	1.83

of capability calculated on the sample. Intuitively, lower sample sizes require higher values of sample $\hat{C}_{pk}$ in order to exceed a minimum threshold and vice versa. Table 5.13 lists the evaluation of Eq. (5.2) for common sample sizes and values of $\hat{C}_{pk}$. From Table 5.13, a sample size of 20 and a sample $\hat{C}_{pk} = 1.5$ would not allow for a conclusion of $C_{pk} > 1.33$, whereas a sample size of 30 and a sample $\hat{C}_{pk} = 1.75$ would allow one to conclude $C_{pk} > 1.33$.

5.4.7 Concluding remarks for power and sample size

The key to making good decisions related to patient safety, package integrity, and stability is a well-designed study that is appropriately powered with the right amount of data. Statistical hypothesis testing and process capability can be used to answer a variety of practical questions related to medical packaging. With appropriate knowledge and planning, experimenters can easily evaluate the feasibility of test plans using the corresponding power and sample size analysis. Careful consideration must be used to create a valid space of scenarios with emphasis on validated test methods and observation of data over relevant sources of variability. Of course, attention to detail in the execution of testing is critical to the generation of data for inference. Adhering to these principles will help ensure package integrity and sterility and consequently patient safety in the medical and pharmaceutical packaging industry.

5.5 New developments

For decades, the key business drivers of cost reduction and improving operational efficiencies have led the pharmaceutical industry to improve packaging materials and components. Providing materials suited to protect sensitive products has been consistently accomplished by building on existing packaging material technologies and the core platforms of structural design. Current global business drivers are still emphasizing cost reductions and efficiency improvements. In addition to these drivers, the increased complexity of pharmaceuticals and biologics, medical devices and combination products, and their accompanying packaging challenges is now creating the need for better solutions, such as a new generation of materials and design platforms. Technology advances for finished product packaging is driving a focused effort to improve manufacturing equipment and operational efficiencies. Historically, new processes and materials in the health-care packaging industry are very slowly adopted. This is largely due to the cost of conversion and a risk adverse mindset which results in a very conservative 'wait and see' approach to adoption of new technologies. This conservative approach may not be acceptable in the future as suppliers increase focus on new technologies to support a rapidly changing health-care market. In some cases, new packaging technologies could be the only way to deliver an important new therapy to a patient. Therefore, it is becoming increasingly important for health-care product manufacturers to revisit the mindset and process of packaging technology conversion to keep pace.

The most critical material performance attribute for packaging complex products is that of barrier performance. While material technology continues to improve properties, such as barrier performance, the need for robust packaging systems and operations continues to grow. Packaging equipment improvements focus on efficiency increases. Some improvements include the reduction of change overtimes and difficulty (from machine to machine, as well as product or format changes on one machine) technology to improve safety, improved line clearance efficiencies, smaller footprints, and self-diagnosing machine problems vs time-consuming troubleshooting. The increase in combination products is driving manufacturing product handling changes such as reduced component exposure to minimize bio-burden and the addition of controlled atmosphere areas. There have been significant advances in package filling technologies which have enabled manufacturers to handle micro dosages and sensitive products (such as biologics) as well as accommodating complex combination products like inhalers.

The area of 'connected health care' is rapidly advancing. An example is an electronic closed system where consistent, direct patient monitoring occurs and based on the monitoring, medication is dispensed to a specific area of the body for maximum effectiveness. Electronic and software technology are the basis for this technology. While electronic componentry has long been a part of medical devices, it is relatively new to packaging materials. The industry has had to adapt by developing packaging to contain the electronic componentry and such advancements as the ability to print electronics on a package or device. Sensor technology can be integrated into packaging to monitor the opening of the package or environmental conditions. It is important to understand if there are any compatibility concerns with the electronic components and the proposed method of sterilization. Knowledge of the method and the ranges and durations of the input parameters is very important for the assessment.

An example of a new system for the integration of a drug and a delivery device is a drinking straw filled with a medication dosage form of pellets; 'XStraw' by Dose Sipping Technologies [96]. The exact dose is contained within the straw that contains a control filter so no medication is wasted. This design is an excellent method to assist children or the elderly with taking their medication. To contain the filled straw, new packaging was developed consisting of polypropylene and an aluminum blister that provide an air tight system which does not require any special storage conditions.

An example of polymer technology evolving to meet the market needs is the development of the family of cyclic olefin homopolymers and copolymers. The family is providing needed performance improvements for several types of health-care product packages. These thermoplastics can be injection molded, extruded, or coextruded to make both rigid or flexible packaging materials. The plastics are inert, pure, safe, and optically clear. Their inert properties make them compatible with gas, steam, and radiation methods of sterilization. These materials offer an excellent alternative to glass vials, bottles, and prefilled glass syringes because of their high optical clarity, excellent moisture barrier properties, and minimal extractables and leachables. Packaging constructed of this material is superior to glass because of its light weight, resistance to breaking, and its elimination of silicone lubricants. The cyclic polyolefins also have found its way into

1. Adhesive systems for medication patches that directly adhere to the patient skin,
2. Packaging that are used in rigid and flexible thermoforming as an alternative to polyethylene terephthalate glycol (PETG) and polyvinyl chloride (PVC) for rigid or flexible thermoforming,

3. Heat sealing layers for devices and pharmaceuticals that do not adsorb or interact with active ingredients, and
4. Other applications such as diagnostics, product mold components, scanning technology, and bone cement mixers for orthopedic procedures [97, 98].

The rapid application of this new material family is an indication of the need for materials with improved performance. New product delivery methods, such as the medication straw, are also needed to safely deliver new biologics and pharmaceuticals. Innovations and the operational developments such as these are necessary to provide safe and effective packaging systems for the increasingly complex combination products [19, 21, 98].

Developments on the technology will not be successful or will be adopted slowly if the regulatory processes do not keep pace. New regulations are increasing the requirements resulting in increased efforts to comply. Regulatory authorities are simultaneously promoting new initiatives to allow patients to have faster access to new innovative devices, while containing or reducing health-care cost. The US FDA CDRH has launched its regulatory science development priorities for improved and faster regulatory decision making in 2017. It includes areas like the modernization of biocompatibility and biological risk evaluation of device materials and reducing Healthcare Associated Infections (HAIs) by better understanding the effectiveness of antimicrobials, sterilization, and reprocessing of medical devices. The idea is also to work collaboratively with external stakeholders to maximize the impact of regulatory science research investments. Science clearly plays a key role, but so do standards. State-of-the-art global consensus standards enhance competition and allow leveraging of regulatory efforts over various regions. Participation of authorities in standard development is also essential. While the US FDA and the authorities of Japan, Canada, Australia, and Brazil are present in key standardization committees, the EU authority's participation recently did not reflect the relative size of the economy. The 2012 EU regulation on European standardization [99] clearly encourages European authorities to participate in TCs as an essential activity required for successful collaboration with industry stakeholders. The new EU MDR [18] continues to build on the "New Legislative Framework" concept based on "harmonized" standards which provide presumption of conformity with essential elements of the law. Harmonization of revised and of new standards, however, has been lagging even under the medical device directives. To prepare for the transition to the new regulatory regime and to improve the situation of harmonized standards, the EU Commission introduced in 2018 a new system with harmonized standards consultants to be involved in the standardization process. The new MDRs [18, 100] also provide the EU Commission with the delegated authority to adopt so-called "common specifications" if standards are not considered sufficient. Despite this new tool, the promotion of consensus standard and the involvement of authorities in the development process will be important for all countries to create the foundation for patient safety and sustainable innovation in the context of a global economy. This is even more critical to countries like India that are in the process of adopting new modern MDRs.

Minimizing packaging waste has long been a focus of various regulations with the objective to minimize landfill and incineration and increase recycling rates that reduce the impact on the environment. The emergence of global climate change initiatives that limits CO_2 and greenhouse gas emissions will likely result in further regulations that will impact the development of products and its packaging. In 2008, ISO and CEN have adopted a guide on addressing environmental issues in product standards [101]. More and more standards with environmental clauses are emerging, such as the 2018 revision of ISO11607. The EU has announced the "Circular Economy" initiative in 2015 [102] with an extensive action plan. The objective is that "*the value of products, materials and resources is maintained in the economy for as long as possible, and the generation of waste [is] minimised,*" so that total carbon dioxide emissions are lowered. These initiatives will shake the status-quo, create new business opportunities, and boost innovation. The entire supply chain including the packaging system designs will have to be reconsidered. *"Life-cycle thinking"* covering all environmental aspects at all stages of a product lifecycle will become an important skill for product and packaging designers and engineers. Targeted technical guides have emerged, like the HPRC Design Guidelines for Optimal Hospital Plastics Recycling [103] published by the Hospital Plastics Recycling Council and TIR65:2015 *Sustainability of medical devices—Elements of a responsible product life cycle* [104] published by AAMI, goes beyond simply addressing waste. Sustainability is indeed a much larger issue that will increasingly drive purchasing decisions, the ability of corporations to attract talent, business ethics and of course business success. All of these will be important drivers and inputs for product and packaging developments in the future.

References

[1] International Organization for Standardization, ISO 11607-1:2006/Amd 1:2014 Packaging for Terminally Sterilized Medical Devices—Part, Vol. 1, Requirements for materials, sterile barrier systems and packaging systems, Geneva, 2014.

[2] International Organization for Standardization, ISO 11607-2:2006/Amd 1:2014 Packaging for Terminally Sterilized Medical Devices—Part, Vol. 2, Validation requirements for forming, sealing and assembly processes, Geneva, 2014.

[3] Sterilization of Medical Products, Kilmer Conference Proceedings, National Conference Center, East Windsor, NJ, 1976.
[4] F.B. Kilmer, Modern Surgical Dressings, Am. J. Pharm. 69 (1897) 15.
[5] Senate and House of Representatives of the United States of America, Medical Device Amendments of 1976, 1976.
[6] Allen, D., Looking back over 20 years of sterile medical packaging (Available at http://www.packagingdigest.com/medical-packaging/looking-back-20-years-of-sterile-medical-pkg-pmp). Pharmaceutical & Medical Packaging News, 2013. January/February 2013.
[7] U.S. Food & Drug Administration (FDA), The Food and Drug Administration's quality system regulations for medical devices (QSRs), Handi-Regs #9603 Keystone Press, Bradenton, FL, 1997, p. 44.
[8] European Committee for Standardization, EN 868-1:1997 Packaging materials and systems for medical devices which are to be sterilized—Part 1. General requirements and test methods. 1997.
[9] European Committee for Standardization, EN 868—Packaging for Terminally Sterilized Medical Devices—Part 2: Sterilization Wrap–Requirements and Test Methods, 2009 (CEN: Brussels).
[10] European Committee for Standardization, EN 868 - Packaging for Terminally Sterilized Medical Devices—Part 3: Paper for Use in the Manufacture of Paper Bags (Specified in EN 868-4) and in the Manufacture of Pouches and Reels (Specified in EN 868-5)—Requirements and Test Methods, 2009 (CEN: Brussels).
[11] European Committee for Standardization, EN 868 - Packaging for Terminally Sterilized Medical Devices—Part 4: Paper Bags—Requirements and Test Methods, 2009 (CEN: Brussels).
[12] European Committee for Standardization, EN 868—Packaging for Terminally Sterilized Medical Devices - Part 6: Paper for Low Temperature Sterilization Processes - Requirements and Test Methods, 2009 (CEN: Brussels).
[13] European Committee for Standardization, EN 868—Packaging for Terminally Sterilized Medical Devices—Part 7: Adhesive Coated Paper for Low Temperature Sterilization Processes—Requirements and Test Methods, 2009 (CEN: Brussels).
[14] European Committee for Standardization, EN 868—Packaging for Terminally Sterilized Medical Devices—Part 8: Re-Usable Sterilization Containers for Steam Sterilizers Conforming to EN 285—Requirements and Test Methods, 2009 (CEN: Brussels).
[15] European Committee for Standardization, EN 868—Packaging for Terminally Sterilized Medical Devices—Part 9: Uncoated Nonwoven Materials of Polyolefines—Requirements and Test Methods, 2009 (CEN: Brussels).
[16] European Committee for Standardization, EN 868 - Packaging for Terminally Sterilized Medical Devices - Part 10: Adhesive Coated Nonwoven Materials of Polyolefines - Requirements and Test Methods, 2009 (CEN: Brussels).
[17] Scholla, M.H., *Medical Packaging: Achieving a Single Global Standard (available at:* http://www.mddionline.com/article/medical-packaging-achieving-single-global-standard), in MDDI. 2004, Can. Underwrit.
[18] Council and European Parliament, Regulation (Eu) 2017/745 of the European Parliament and of the Council of 5 April 2017 on medical devices, amending Directive 2001/83/EC, Regulation (EC) No 178/2002 and Regulation (EC) No 1223/2009 and repealing Council Directives 90/385/EEC and 93/42/EEC, in *2017/745*, 2017. Brussels.
[19] M. Barbella, Artful adaption: packaging and sterilization providers must keep pace with rapid change to innovate, grow and improve safety., in Medical Product Outsourcing, Rodman Publishing, 2014 (The: The Free Library).
[20] D. Allen, Combination products: What role does packaging play? in: Pharmaceutical & Medical Packaging News, 2015.
[21] M.P. Drues, Combination Products 101: A Primer For Medical Device Makers, in Med Device Online, 2014, pp. 1–4.

[22] J. Wiley, The Wiley Encyclopedia of Packaging Technology, John Wiley & Sons, New York, NY USA; Toronto, Canada, 1986, p. 746.
[23] United States Pharmacopoeia (USP/NF), USP 34 General Notices and Requirements. 2011.
[24] U.S. Food & Drug Administration (FDA), Guidance for Industry—Container Closure Systems for Packaging Human Drugs and Biologics—Chemistry, Manufacturing, and Controls Documentation (http://www.fda.gov/downloads/Drugs/.../Guidances/ucm070551.pdf). 1999: Rockville, Maryland.
[25] U.S. Food & Drug Administration (FDA), Applying Human Factors and Usability Engineering to Medical Devices—Guidance for Industry and Food and Drug Administration Staff, Center for Devices and Radiological Health (CDRH), Editor. 2016.
[26] U.S. Food & Drug Administration (FDA), Draft Guidance—Human Factors Studies and Related Clinical Study Considerations in Combination Product Design and Development, Center for Devices and Radiological Health, et al., Editors. 2016.
[27] Sterile Barrier Association, Compatibility of Materials Used for Sterile Barrier Systems with Sterilisation Processes, [cited 2017 11 July 2017]; Available from: http://www.sterilebarrier.org/media/22919/Sterilisation-compatibility.pdf, 2010.
[28] United States Pharmacopoeia (USP/NF), Chapter <797> Pharmaceutical compounding sterile preparations, in: Chapter <797>. 2016, accessed.
[29] R.J. Hernandez, S.E.M. Selke, J.D. Culter, Plastics Packaging (Properties, Processing, Applications, and Regulations), ed. H.P.H.G. Publishers, Vol. 1, Munich, Germany; Cincinnati, Ohio, Hanser Publishers; Hanser Gardner Publishers, 2000. 425.
[30] J.D. O'Brien, M. Sherman, Medical Device Packaging Handbook, second ed., Marcel Dekker, 1998.
[31] U.S. Food & Drug Administration (FDA). Frequently Asked Questions About Combination Products. 2016; Available from: http://www.fda.gov/CombinationProducts/AboutCombinationProducts/ucm101496.htm.
[32] U.S. Food & Drug Administration (FDA), Early Development Considerations for Innovative Combination Products (http://www.fda.gov/downloads/RegulatoryInformation/Guidances/ucm126054.pdf), in Office of Combination Products-Guidance for Industry. 2011.
[33]. U.S. Food & Drug Administration (FDA), Draft-Guidance for Industry-Current Good Manufacturing Practice Requirements for Combination Products, U.S. Department of Health and Human Services, et al., Editors. 2013.
[34] U.S. Food & Drug Administration (FDA), 21 CFR—Chapter I-Food & Drug Administration-Department of Health and Human Services-Subchapter H—Medical Devices—Part 820 Quality System Regulation (http://www.ecfr.gov/cgi-bin/text-idx?SID=39df3a74818e54ae1ca405f599ac630f&mc=true&node=pt21.8.820&rgn=div5). 2016.
[35] International Organization for Standardization, ISO 13485:2016—Medical devices—Quality management systems—Requirements for regulatory purposes. 2016: Geneva.
[36] European Committee for Standardization, EN ISO 11607-1:2009/Amd 1:2014 Packaging for Terminally Sterilized Medical Devices—Part, Vol. 1, Requirements for materials, sterile barrier systems and packaging systems, Brussels, Geneva, 2014.
[37] ASTM International, F2097-10 Standard guide for design and evaluation of primary flexible packaging for medical products. 2010: West Conshohocken, PA 19428-2959, United States.
[38] International Organization for Standardization, ISO/TS 16775 Packaging for Terminally Sterilized Medical Devices - Guidance on the Application of ISO 11607-1 and ISO 11607-2, 2014.
[39] United States Pharmacopoeia (USP/NF), USP <1207> Sterile Product Packaging—Integrity Evaluation.

[40] L.S. Burrell, et al., Development of a dye ingress method to assess container-closure integrity: Correlation to microbial ingress, PDA J. Pharm. Sci. Technol. 54 (6) (2000) 449–455.
[41] Keller, S., Determination of the leak size critical to package sterility maintenance, in *Food Science and Technology*. 1998, Faculty of Virginia Polytechnic Institute and State University: Blacksburg, Virginia. p. 191.
[42] M.J. Akers, Sterile Drug Products: Formulation, Packaging, Manufacturing, and Quality, Informa Healthcare. ix, New York, 2010, p. 505.
[43] E.T. Hackett, et al., How small is small? The effects of pinholes on medical packaging, Medical Device and Diagnostic Industry 22 (8) (2000) 52–66.
[44] ASTM International, F1886/F1886M—09 Standard Test Method for Determining Integrity of Seals for Flexible Packaging by Visual Inspection. 2009: West Conshohocken, PA 19428-2959, United States.
[45] ASTM International, ASTM F1929-15 Standard Test Method for Detecting Seal Leaks in Porous Medical Packaging by Dye Penetration, 2015 (West Conshohocken - PA 19428-2959, United States).
[46] ASTM International, F2096-11 Standard Test Method for Detecting Gross Leaks in Packaging by Internal Pressurization (Bubble Test). 2011: West Conshohocken, PA.
[47] ASTM International, ASTM F2338-09(2013)—Standard Test Method for Nondestructive Detection of Leaks in Packages by Vacuum Decay Method. 2013, ASTM International.
[48] ASTM International, ASTM F3004-13e1—Standard Test Method for Evaluation of Seal Quality and Integrity Using Airborne Ultrasound. 2013, ASTM International.
[49] L. Jones, et al., Quest of Sterile Packaging: Part I—Approaches to Package Testing, Medical Device and Diagnostic Industry, 1995.
[50] J. Hansen, et al., Quest of Sterile Packaging: Part II—Physical Package Integrity Test Methods, Medical Device and Diagnostic Industry, 1995.
[51] A. Tallentire, C.S. Sinclair, Discriminating method for measuring the microbial barrier performance of medical packaging papers, Vol. 18, Medical Device and Diagnostic Industry, 1996, p. 5.
[52] C.S. Sinclair, A. Tallentire, Definition of a correlation between microbiological and physical particulate barrier performances for porous medical packaging materials, PDA J. Pharm. Sci. Technol. 56 (1) (2002) 11–19.
[53] ASTM International, ASTM F2638-12e1—Standard Test Method for Using Aerosol Filtration for Measuring the Performance of Porous Packaging Materials as a Surrogate Microbial Barrier, 2016.
[54] P. Herman, C. Larsen, Measuring Porous Microbial Barriers—Part I & II, MDDI, 2008.
[55] Wagner, T., ASTM F2638 Test Method, Porous Packaging Materials & Microbial Barrier Performance (*h*ttps://www.packagingdigest.com/testing/pmp-astm-f2638-test-method-porous-packaging-materials-microbial-barrier-performance-130225). Pharmaceutical & Medical Packaging News, 2013.
[56] H. Dunkelberg, U. Schmelz, Determination of the efficacy of sterile barrier systems against microbial challenges during transport and storage, Infect. Control Hosp. Epidemiol. 30 (2) (2009) 179–183.
[57] H. Dunkelberg, F. Fleitmann-Glende, Measurement of the microbial barrier effectiveness of sterilization containers in terms of the log reduction value for prevention of nosocomial infections, Am. J. Infect. Control 34 (5) (2006) 285–289.
[58] H. Dunkelberg, S. Rohmann, Test to determine sterile integrity of wrapped medical products at a probability of recontamination of 1:1,000,000, Infect. Control Hosp. Epidemiol. 27 (4) (2006) 367–371.
[59] J. Severin, et al., A new methodology for whole-package microbial challenge testing for medical device trays, J. Test. Eval. 35 (4) (2007) 373–380.

[60] ASTM International, F88/F88M-09 Standard Test Method for Seal Strength of Flexible Barrier Materials. 2009:West Conshohocken, PA 19428-2959, United States.

[61] European Committee for Standardization, EN 868 - Packaging for Terminally Sterilized Medical Devices—Part 5: Sealable Pouches and Reels of Porous Materials and Plastic Film Construction—Requirements and Test Methods, 2009 (CEN: Brussels).

[62] European Commission, EudraLex—Volume 4—EU Guidelines for Good Manufacturing Practice for Medicinal Products for Human and Veterinary Use—Annex 15: Qualification and Validation, Directorate-General for Health and Food Safety, Editor, 2015. Brussels.

[63] International Council for Harmonisation (ICH), Validation of Analytical Procedures: Text and Methodology Q2(R1), 2005.

[64] ASTM International, *ASTM E691–15 Standard Practice for Conducting an Interlaboratory Study to Determine the Precision of a Test Method.* 2015, ASTM International.

[65] International Organization for Standardization, ISO 5725-1:1994 Accuracy (Trueness and Precision) of Measurement Methods and Results—Part, Vol. 1, General principles and definitions, Geneva, 1994.

[66] International Organization for Standardization, ISO 5725-2:1994 Accuracy (trueness and precision) of measurement methods and results—Part 2: Basic method for the determination of repeatability and reproducibility of a standard measurement method. 1994.

[67] Council and European Parliament, Proposal for a REGULATION OF THE EUROPEAN PARLIAMENT AND OF THE COUNCIL on Medical Devices, and Amending Directive 2001/83/EC, Regulation (EC) no 178/2002 and Regulation (EC) no 1223/2009. 2016.

[68] International Organization for Standardization, ISO 10993-1:2009—Biological Evaluation of Medical Devices—Part Vol. 1: Evaluation and testing within a risk management process. 2009: Geneva.

[69] ASTM International, ASTM F2475-11 Standard Guide for Biocompatibility Evaluation of Medical Device Packaging Materials, 2011.

[70] S.C. Gad, M.G. McCord, S.C. Gad, Safety Evaluation in the Development of Medical Devices and Combination Products, third ed., Informa Healthcare, New York, 2008, p. 300. viii.

[71] European Medicine Agency (EMA), EMA Guideline on Plastic Immediate Packaging Materials, in CPMP/QWP/4359/03 and EMEA/CVMP/205/04, C.F.M.P.F.H.U. (CHMP) and C.F.M.P.F.V.U. (CVMP), Editors. 2005: London.

[72] International Organization for Standardization, ISO 11607-1:2009/Amd 1:2014 Packaging for Terminally Sterilized Medical Devices—Part, Vol. 1, Requirements for materials, sterile barrier systems and packaging systems, Geneva, 2014.

[73] D4169-09 standard practice for performance testing of shipping containers and systems, in: ASTM International, 2009. West Conshohocken, PA 19428-2959, United States.

[74] ISTA, Guidelines for selecting and using ISTA® test procedures & projects. 2012.

[75] international Organization for Standardization, ISO 11139 Sterilization of Health Care Products—Vocabulary of Terms Used in Sterilization and Related Equipment and Process Standards, 2018. Geneva.

[76] T. Trier, et al., The role of packaging size on contamination rates during simulated presentation to a sterile field, PLoS One 9 (7) (2014).

[77] SBA, Usability of sterile barrier systems for medical devices, Sterile Barrier Association (SBA), 2015.

[78] European Commission, Commission Communication in the Framework of the Implementation of the Council Directive 93/42/EEC Concerning Medical Devices (Text with EEA Relevance) (Publication of Titles and References of Harmonised Standards under the Directive). OJ, 2009. C 41/06.

[79] Council, COUNCIL DIRECTIVE of 20 June 1990 on the approximation of the laws of the Member States relating to active implantable medical devices (90/385/EEC) as amended by Council Directive 93/42/EEC of 14 June 1993, Council Directive 93/68/EEC of 22 July 1993, Regulation (EC) No 1882/2003 of the European Parliament and of the Council of 29 September 2003 and by Directive 2007/47/EC of the European Parliament and of the Council of 5 September 2007 (consolidated version). OJ, 1990. L 189.
[80] Council and European Parliament, DIRECTIVE 2001/83/EC OF THE EUROPEAN PARLIAMENT AND OF THE COUNCIL of 6 November 2001 on the Community code relating to medicinal products for human use. OJ, 2001. L 311, 28.11.2001, p. 67.
[81] ASTM International, F1980—16 Standard Guide for Accelerated Aging of Sterile Barrier Systems for Medical Devices, 2016. West Conshohocken, PA 19428-2959, United States.
[82] U.S. Food & Drug Administration (FDA), 21 CFR-Chapter I-Subchapter C-Part 211—Current Good Manufacturing Practice for Finished Pharmaceuticals, in 21. 2016.
[83] International Council for Harmonisation (ICH), ICH Quality Guidelines, http://www.ich.org/products/guidelines/quality/article/quality-guidelines.html.
[84] International Council for Harmonisation (ICH), ICH Harmonised Tripartite Guideline—Stability Testing of New Drug Substances and Products Q1A(R2). 2003.
[85] Global Harmonization Task Force, GHTF-SG3—Quality Management Systems—Process Validation Guidance. 2004.
[86] U.S. Food & Drug Administration (FDA), Guidance for Industry—Process Validation: General Principles and Practices (http://www.fda.gov/downloads/Drugs/Guidance-ComplianceRegulatoryInformation/Guidances/UCM070336.pdf), Center for Drug Evaluation and Research (CDER), Center for Biologics Evaluation and Research (CBER), and Center for Veterinary Medicine (CVM), Editors. 2011.
[87] Notified Body Operations Group (NBOG), ed, NBOG BPG 2014-3—Guidance for Manufacturers and Notified Bodies on Reporting of Design Changes and Changes of the Quality System, European Association for Medical Devices of Notified Bodies, Brussels, 2014.
[88] T. Wagner, M.H. Scholla, Sterile barrier systems: managing changes and revalidations, http://www.ivtnetwork.com/article/sterile-barrier-systems-managing-changes-and-revalidations. J. Validation Technol. 19 (3) (2013).
[89] N. Kaller, Medical Packaging Study—Reducing the Risk of Failure through Performance Testing of Packaging Made from Various Materials, Medical Packaging Community, DuPont, 2014, p. 22.
[90] Sterile Barrier Association, Sample Validation Flow Diagram, [cited 2017 6 July 2017]; Available from: http://www.sterilebarrier.org/medical-device-manufacturers/validation-process/sample-validation-flow-diagram/, 2017.
[91] D.S. Moore, W.I. Notz, M.A. Fligner, The Basic Practice of Statistics, Macmillan Learning, 2015.
[92] J. Stein, N. Doganaksoy, Sample size considerations for assessing the equivalence of two process means, Qual. Eng. 12 (1) (1999) 105–110.
[93] D.J. Schuirmann, A comparison of the two one-sided tests procedure and the power approach for assessing the equivalence of average bioavailability, J. Pharmacokinet. Biopharm. 15 (6) (1987) 657–680.
[94] L.S. Nelson, Nomograph of sample size for estimating standard deviation, J. Qual. Technol. 8 (3) (1976) 179–180.
[95] D.C. Montgomery, Introduction to Statistical Quality Control, J. Wiley & Sons, 2013.
[96] E. Sternberger-Rutzel, Drinking Medicines with a Straw Instead of Swallowing 'bitter' Pills, 2014.

[97] J. Cui, et al., Synthesis of High Performance Cyclic Olefin Polymers (COPS) with Ester Group via Ring-Opening Metathesis Polymerization, in: Polymers, 2015, p. 31.
[98] J.H. Schut, New cyclic olefins, in: Plastics Technology, 2000.
[99] Parliament, E. and Council, REGULATION (EU) No 1025/2012 of 25 October 2012 on European standardisation, amending Council Directives 89/686/EEC and 93/15/EEC and Directives 94/9/EC, 94/25/EC, 95/16/EC, 97/23/EC, 98/34/EC, 2004/22/EC, 2007/23/EC, 2009/23/EC and 2009/105/EC of the European Parliament and of the Council and repealing Council Decision 87/95/EEC and Decision No 1673/2006/EC of the European Parliament and of the Council, in 1025/2012, European Union, Editor. 2012: Brussels.
[100] Council and European Parliament, REGULATION (EU) 2017/746 OF THE EUROPEAN PARLIAMENT AND OF THE COUNCIL of 5 April 2017 on In Vitro Diagnostic Medical Devices and Repealing Directive 98/79/EC and Commission Decision 2010/227/EU. 2017: Brussels.
[101] International Organization for Standardization, ISO Guide 64:2008—Guide for addressing environmental issues in product standards. 2008: Geneva.
[102] European Commission, Communication From The Commission to the European Parliament, the Council, The European Economic And Social Committee And The Committee Of The Regions—Closing the loop—An EU action plan for the Circular Economy. 2015: Brussels.
[103] Healthcare Plastics Recycling Council, HPRC—Design Guidelines for Optimal Hospital Plastics Recycling. 2016.
[104] AAMI, TIR65:2015—Sustainability of medical devices—Elements of a responsible product life cycle. 2015, AAMI.

CHAPTER 6

Review of current practice in preventing health care associated infections

Donna Swenson[a]
AAMI, Arlington, VA, United States

Contents

6.1 Introduction

Health-care-associated infections (HAIs) are a major global problem and can be caused by many factors including: improper cleaning, inadequate sterilization, and improper handling of medical devices. It is difficult to determine the cause of an HAI because the infections are diagnosed days after the procedure. There is, however, growing evidence that improper health-care professional practices play a significant factor in the occurrence

[a]Independent expert in medical device sterilization.

Assurance of Sterility for Sensitive Combination Products and Materials
https://doi.org/10.1016/B978-0-12-805082-8.00006-2

of HAIs. Although single-use medical devices have not traditionally been a major source of infection, great strides have recently been made in treating and preventing these types of HAIs.

6.2 Background in HAIs

HAIs affect patients or staff who are or were in a health-care facility (HCF) but the infection was not present or incubating at the time of admission or work. These include infections that were acquired at the HCF but that did not appear until after discharge. Occupational infections among HCF staff are also counted in HAIs.

HAIs are currently the most common adverse event that occurs in health-care delivery worldwide. In developed countries 7 of every 100 hospital patients will acquire at least one HAI while in the hospital. In developing countries, 10 of every 100 patients will get an HAI. Each year in the United States, 2 million people in HCFs will acquire serious infections from bacteria that are resistant to one or more antimicrobial agents. Of these 2 million people, approximately 23,000 people will die as a result of these infections. Even more people will die from other conditions that were complicated by an HAI [1].

HAIs are a problem globally in all areas of the hospital. Data from 2002 show that on average in the European Union (EU) the average HAI rate was 7.1% and in the United States the average was 4.5% [2]. The rate changes significantly according to the procedure and the condition of the patient. ICU patients have the highest incidence of infections and are associated primarily with invasive medical devices, e.g., central venous lines, urinary catheters, and ventilators. Newborns are another higher-risk patient population. Surgical site infections (SSIs) are also a significant problem especially in developing countries. Up to 30% of intensive care unit (ICU) patients in developed countries will get at least one HAI. The rate of infections can jump to 66% of patients with surgery in developing countries.

HAIs are widespread, and events are under reported because many countries do not have effective surveillance systems. HAIs are frequently hidden from the public's view except when high-profile incidents occur, which capture media attention. The recent duodenoscope infections due to re-cleaning challenges and cross infection of Ebola are prime examples of this, but even these events quickly lose the public interest. No institution or country can claim to have solved the problem of HAIs.

6.3 Assessment of risk

There are many risk factors that contribute to the development of HAIs. Prolonged and/or inappropriate use of invasive devices as well as antibiotics has created a major problem. There is an increased probability that an infection will occur if there is a breach in the skin barrier or the longer an invasive device is in place. Examples of this are the use of intravenous or urinary catheters or whenever surgery is performed. With new treatment options becoming available, procedures today can be more complex, sophisticated, and use more devices. These factors combine to increase the probability of an infection occurring. In addition to these factors, treatments are available for patients who have more health issues that make them prone to getting an HAI. Patients have comorbidities such as diabetes and high blood pressure, or are on immunosuppressants which also increase the risk of infection.

In addition to these patient-related factors there are resource factors that can increase the potential for a patient to get an HAI. Poor infrastructure including poor environmental hygiene and waste disposal can increase the occurrence of HAIs. Inadequate staffing will result in the tendency of health-care workers to skip steps and to work faster than is safe. Infection control procedures require a meticulous attention to details. Skipping steps or performing those steps too quickly can result in problems. For example, medical device manufacturers provide step-by-step instructions for cleaning reusable devices. It is well known that many times these instructions are not followed exactly. On September 11 2015, the US FDA and CDC issued a joint CDC Health Advisory to alert all US hospitals that there was an immediate need for HCFs to review procedures for cleaning, disinfecting, and sterilizing reusable medical devices. In this alert, it was stated that "recent infection control lapses due to noncompliance with recommended reprocessing procedures highlight a critical gap in patient safety" [3]. Staff at some HCFs have been poorly trained in basic infection control practices and do not have adequate knowledge of how to do their jobs. This is particularly true in ancillary support service departments such as environmental services and sterile processing. In addition to inadequate training, many facilities lack standard procedures. Procedures need to be standardized to ensure a consistent quality service. It is not possible to evaluate the quality of the department's services when different employees are providing the same service or product in different ways. In September 2016, a forum on Medical Technology and HAIs was held. This meeting was a collaboration of AAMI, AHA, CDC, FDA/CDRH, and the Joint Commission. The purpose of this forum was to work toward developing solutions to prevent device-associated HAIs. Specifically, the attendees looked at causes and solutions in terms of three factors: people, places, and things.

There is also an issue with the underreporting of HAIs. Many HAIs are not diagnosed until after the patients are discharged because hospital stays are shorter than the incubation time for a pathogenic organism to cause an infection. Any infection that becomes evident within 48 h after hospitalization is considered an HAI. However, many SSIs do not exhibit symptoms until around 21 days after surgery and some organisms have much longer incubation times meaning that these infections may not be counted as an HAI.

6.3.1 Identifying HAIs

The CDC defines an HAI as a localized or systemic condition resulting from an adverse reaction to the presence of an infectious agent(s) or its toxin(s). To be classified as an HAI, there must be no evidence that the infection was present or incubating at the time of admission to the acute care setting, indicating that if the patient gets an infection while at the HCF then the infection was acquired in the HCF and is an HAI [4]. HAIs can originate from endogenous sources (body sites such as skin, nose, mouth, GI tract, vagina) or from exogenous sources (eternal to the patience such as other personnel, equipment, medical devices, or the health-care. Infections in infants that result from passage through the birth canal are included in HAIs.

However, many infections that a patient in the hospital has are not considered an HAI. These include the following:

- infections that were present when the patient was admitted to the HCF,
- infections in infants acquired transplacentally, e.g., herpes simplex, syphilis and that become evident within 48 h of delivery,
- reactivation of a latent infection, e.g., herpes zoster (shingles), syphilis, and tuberculosis (TB),
- colonization of microorganisms on skin, mucous membranes in open wounds or in excretions or secretions but not causing adverse clinical signs or symptoms, and
- inflammation that results from tissue response to injury or stimulation by noninfectious agents, e.g., chemicals.

6.3.2 Assessing the burden/impact of HAIs

HAIs pose a significant impact to the patient, their family, and on society. Patients are subject to additional pain and suffering such as fever and prolonged hospital stays. An HAI can lead to further issues including long-term disability and even death. There is a huge financial burden for HCFs with the overall direct cost ranging from $1006 to $25,546 for a single US Hospital HAI.

In addition to the direct financial impact on the HCF, it is estimated that HAIs cost 7 billion euros in the EU and 6.5 billion dollars in the United States in lost productivity. The HAI Prevalence Survey results were published in 2014 which described the burden of HAIs in US hospitals. The survey reported that in 2011, there were an estimated 721,800 HAIs in US acute-care hospitals. These consisted of the following types and numbers [5]:

- Pneumonia: 157,500
- SSIs, inpatient surgery: 157,500
- Gastrointestinal illness: 123,100
- Urinary tract infections: 93,300
- Primary bloodstream infections: 71,900

About 75,000 patients with HAIs died during their hospitalizations. Additional HAIs occurred due to other reasons not cited in this report. Limitations in scope and data collection methods preclude data from various studies providing complete information on national rates of HAIs. For this reason, estimates from different studies will differ.

6.4 Causes of HAIs

Leadership is an important component in preventing HAIs. Senior leadership needs to promote a culture of safety. Though this may sound simple, it is not that easy to do. Processes need to be developed to ensure that employees can report and openly discuss safety without fear of retaliation and intimidation. According to the 2016 Hospital Survey on Patient Safety Culture by the Agency for Healthcare Research and Quality (AHRQ), there are several areas where hospitals need to improve in the culture of safety [6]. In the User Comparative Database from this report, the average percent positive responses range from 82% to 45%. Composite topics are shown below in order from highest average percent positive response to the lowest.

- Teamwork Within Units
- Supervisor/Manager Expectations and Actions Promoting Patient Safety
- Organizational Learning—Continuous Improvement
- Management Support for Patient Safety
- Feedback and Communication About Error
- Frequency of Events Reported
- Overall Perceptions of Patient Safety

- Communication Openness
- Teamwork Across Units
- Staffing
- Handoffs and Transitions
- Nonpunitive Response to Error

In 2005, WHO launched a Global Patient Safety Challenge, "Clean Care Is Safer Care." This initiative targeted the reduction of HAIs by promoting best hand hygiene practices. The ongoing vision is to make all aspects of infection prevention and control a priority for global health care. Ten years of "Clean Care is Safer Care" has saved millions of lives and has prevented infections in both patients and HCWs [7].

Following closely behind hand hygiene as a method of preventing infections is environmental cleanliness. It is important that terminal cleaning is performed daily in patient care areas as well as areas where contamination is a higher risk, e.g., patient rooms, surgery operating rooms, and sterile processing decontamination rooms. Terminal cleaning needs to be performed with a germicide labeled for standard cleaning and disinfection. Quaternary ammonium compounds are the most frequently used to disinfect environmental surfaces. Hypochlorite-based product (bleach) must be used for known *Clostridium difficile (C. diff)* patient room cleaning. Bleach products degrade quickly so they usually cannot be made in advance. Some practitioners prefer to use bleach wipes for this reason. When a patient is in contact isolation, disposable patient care items should be used as a precaution. Environmental cleaning is important as a means of preventing infection transmission by indirect contact.

CDC publishes an annual HAI Progress Report that details the current state in controlling HAIs on several important criteria. According to the CDCs annual HAI Progress Report published in 2016 (data from 2014):

1. There was a 50% decrease in central line-associated blood stream infections (CLABSIs) between 2008 and 2014. A central line is a type of catheter that is placed in a large vein that allows multiple IV fluids to be given and blood to be drawn. A central line catheter is a thin tube, but it's much longer than a regular IV tube.
2. There was no change in overall catheter-associated urinary tract infections (CAUTIs) rates between 2009 and 2014.
3. There was progress in non-ICU settings for CAUTIs between 2009 and 2014, and in all settings between 2013 and 2014 and even more progress in all settings toward the end of 2014.
4. There was a 17% decrease in SSIs related to the 10 select procedures tracked (hip arthroplasty, knee arthroplasty, colon surgery, rectal surgery,

abdominal hysterectomy, vaginal hysterectomy, coronary artery bypass graft, other cardiac surgery, peripheral vascular bypass surgery, and abdominal aortic aneurysm repair).

5. There was an 8% decrease in hospital-onset *C diff* infections between 2011 and 2014.
6. There was a 13% decrease in hospital-onset methicillin-resistant *Staphylococcus aureus* (MRSA) bacteremia between 2011 and 2014 [8].

Steps can be taken to control and prevent HAIs from occurring. It has been shown that specific target HAIs can be decreased by as much as 70% when HCF teams are aware of infection problems and take specific steps to prevent infections. Preventing HAIs is possible, but it takes a conscious effort of everyone involved in the patient's care to address the issue. A successful program to address preventing HAIs requires a systematic approach: the health-care facilities, their employees, public health, quality improvement groups, the Federal Government, and the patient all working together. See section on Preventing HAIs later in this chapter for additional information on steps that can be taken to prevent HAIs from occurring.

6.4.1 Patient-related factors

Several patient-related factors need to be considered when looking at how diseases are transmitted. Many factors including patient characteristics, influence whether an infectious disease will be transmitted to a person. Infectious disease transmission can be thought of as a chain with each link in the chain needed before the infection will be transmitted. Each of the following links must be present before an infection can be transmitted:

- Source of microorganisms
- Susceptible host and
- Means of transmission

There are several ways to break each of these links in disease transmission. Steps can be taken to remove the source of microorganisms. People can improve nutrition, get exercise, and get sufficient sleep to improve their immune systems and reduce their susceptibility as a host. Personal protective equipment can be used to prevent patients from being exposed as well as health-care workers and others exposing the patient to new microbes.

6.4.1.1 Source of microorganisms

People are a major source of microorganisms which are a part of a person's normal body flora. Most of these organisms are necessary for each of us to live and be healthy. However, it is also possible for pathogenic microorganisms to colonize on a patient. Infections can be transmitted from other patients, from health-care personnel, from visitors, or from a patient's own body flora. In addition to people, transmission of infection can be from contaminated surfaces or objects, e.g., surgical instrumentation, contaminated surfaces in patient rooms, and contaminated water sources (ice machines).

6.4.1.2 Susceptible host

Even if a source of infectious microorganisms is presented to a host, it does not mean that an infection will result. The host must be susceptible to the infection. There are several intrinsic factors that predispose a patient to infection. The first hurdle is the host's natural skin barrier. Breaching the integrity of the skin increases the chances of getting an infection. Medical and surgical treatment can make a person more likely to get an infection. Next, the infection must overcome the host immune system. Neonates and the elderly tend to have poorly developed or weakened immune systems and thus are more prone to getting an infection. Similarly, hosts with an underlying disease or who are immunocompromised are more likely to succumb to an infection if exposed to microorganisms.

Host factors can impact how quickly or even if HAIs can be eradicated by the host. The host's genetic make-up influences the host's susceptibility to microorganisms. People with certain diseases, e.g., diabetes, will have a more difficult time fighting an infection. Host defenses include:

1. Natural barriers, e.g., intact skin and mucous membranes;
2. Nonspecific immune response, e.g., phagocytic cells (neutrophils, macrophages) and their products; and
3. Specific immune responses, e.g., antibodies, lymphocytes and
4. Natural flora

Intact skin prevents microorganisms from entering sterile body areas. Mucous membranes also provide a barrier to the invasion of microorganisms. In addition, mucous membranes have some antimicrobial properties. The respiratory tract has upper airway filters and coughing can help propel microorganisms away from the respiratory tract out of the body.

An inflammatory response directs the immune system to injury or infection sites. Microbial spread can be limited by inactivation of microorganisms by ingestion by the phagocytes creating a foreign body occlusion. Once ingested, oxidative products produced by the phagocytes will kill microorganisms.

A host can produce a variety of antibodies in response to a specific foreign body response. These antibodies can attract the host's white blood cells (WBCs) and activate the complement system. This can destroy the cell walls of infecting microorganisms.

Today many microorganisms are resistant to the medications that have traditionally been used to treat the infections. This problem has been attributed to overprescribing of antibiotics, poor patient compliance in taking the antibiotics and the ability of bacteria to develop resistance mechanisms through genetic alterations. It has been estimated that up to 50% of antibiotics used in hospitals are used inappropriately [9]. Multidrug-resistant organisms (MDROs) can cause infections in the blood, organ systems, and on skin. MDRO infections have arisen because of over prediction and misuse of antibiotics. As microorganisms are repeatedly exposed to a low dose of a particular antibiotic, they have developed mechanisms that help them to fight the antibiotic. Failure to take antibiotics as prescribed has enabled organisms to develop resistance. Patients often stop taking the prescribed antibiotic as soon as they feel better. The premature stoppage of the antibiotics allows the more difficult to kill microorganisms to survive and results in the microbial population developing a resistance. It is critical that patients complete the regimen of prescribed medication despite the fact that they are feeling better. The probability of the microbe developing resistance increases with the exposure to antibiotics. Once developed, the resistance to the antibiotic can be passed on to new bacteria.

There are some basic steps that can be taken to prevent antibiotic-resistant infections. These include:

- Control of antibiotic use
  - Overuse of antibiotics is a major cause of antibiotic-resistant organisms. Antibiotics, often prescribed for viral infections, only increase the exposure of the microbial population to the antibiotic because antibiotics are not effective against viruses.
  - Use of antibiotics should be targeted for specific bacterial infections. Certain bacteria are more susceptible to specific antibiotics.
  - Antibiotics must be taken as prescribed. The incredible efficacy of antibiotics often lead to rapid symptomatic relief before the bacteria has been eradicated. This leads patients to stop or miss prescribed dosages because they feel better. The resultant exposure of a low residual antibiotic dose to the remaining bacteria which are more difficult to kill, is a perfect storm to develop antibiotic-resistant strains of bacteria.
  - Increased use of antibiotics in an environment where antimicrobial-resistant bacterium already exists provides natural selective pressure to enable these agents to flourish.

- Control of direct person-to-person spread of bacteria
  - MRSA and vancomycin-resistant enterobacter (VRE) are spread primarily by person-to-person contact.
  - Diligent hand washing is needed to prevent spreading bacteria from one place to another. Hands can act as a vehicle for moving bacteria from one location to another and from one person to another.
- Control of indirect person to person spread of microbes
  - Effective cleaning of floors, sinks and other surfaces is needed to minimize the spread of microbes.
  - Effective cleaning of patient care equipment will help to prevent patient to patient transmission of microbes.
  - Surgical instruments and medical devices must be effectively cleaned, disinfected, and/or sterilized. It is important to disinfect surgical instrumentation to prevent transmission to health-care personnel as well as to prevent transmission from one patient to another. A reminder of the importance of cleaning is seen in the recent problems in the United States that resulted in infections from the use of contaminated duodenoscopes.
  - Reducing hospital stays will reduce the potential for exposure to microorganisms that are present on other people.
  - Utilizing outpatient procedures whenever possible will also minimize the potential for patient-to-patient exposure to and transmission of infectious agents.
  - Risk-based personal protective equipment is used to provide protection from infections without raising health-care costs to a point where the cost is prohibitive. For example, AAMI Level 4 protection surgical gowns are only used for procedures where there is expected to be a high volume of blood and other body fluids, e.g., total joint surgery. This level of protection is not needed for surgical procedures where small volumes of blood and body fluid are expected to be present, e.g., eye surgery.

6.4.1.3 Means of transmission

There are many methods by which microorganisms can move from one place to another. Microorganisms can move by direct or indirect contact. Respiratory droplets can occur from coughing, sneezing, talking, suctioning, and during bronchoscopy procedures. The droplets can land on a mucosal surface such as the nose, mouth, or eyes or compromised skin. Transmission can also occur when droplets land on a surface of an inanimate or animate object and then are transferred to a mucosal surface.

Microorganisms can become airborne and become suspended in the air for long periods of time. Air currents will then move these organisms about. This will only happen with small-particle size organisms. Invasive devices provide a portal of entry and facilitate the transfer of microorganisms from one part of the body to another and from the health-care worker to the patient.

A final means of transmitting microorganisms is through a common vehicle. In this transmission method, a common inanimate vehicle of contaminated food, water, medication, solution, device, or equipment can result in a large number of exposures in a short period of time.

6.4.2 Procedural-related characteristics

In addition to the patient-related characteristics there are many procedural characteristics that create a risk for getting an HAI. Patient care variables for procedures include antibiotic use, invasive medical device use, prophylaxis, and patient length of stay (LOS). Administrative variables for procedures include the ratio of nurses to patients, the level of patient care personnel education, use of permanent versus temporary staff, variable use of aseptic techniques used by HCWs, contaminated ventilation and water systems, and the physical layout of the patient care area.

6.4.2.1 Risks based on the procedure

Intact skin is one of our biggest defenses to infection and when the skin is breached it is easier for pathogenic microorganisms to start an infection. The risk of infection increases any time that a surgical or other invasive procedure is performed where the skin is breached. Procedures that involve contact with intact mucous membrane, e.g., endoscopic procedures, carry a lower level of risk compared to procedures that invade sterile areas of the body. The type of procedure being performed will impact the risk of a patient getting an HAI. Any procedure where the skin is breached and normally sterile tissue or the vascular system is invaded carry a higher risk of an HAI occurring.

Even when the skin is not breached, devices that remain in place increase the likelihood of infection, e.g., urinary catheters, ventilators. The chronic nature can lead to abrasion in the skin barrier resulting in a path for microbes to invade the body.

HAI classification

HAIs can be non-device associated or medical device associated. Non-device-associated HAI are predominantly human sources, e.g., patients,

HCWs, household members, and other visitors. Non-device-associated infection can include: SARS, flu, hepatitis B and C, fungal infections from the environment, Noro virus, and Ebola. Standard precautions and respiratory precautions are used to fight transmission of these infections.

Device-associated infections result from the interface of microorganisms with the device and host factors. Although the most important pathogenic factor is the microorganism, device factors are more commonly addressed because of the ability to control them. It is important to understand the different types of HAIs that can occur if we are to effectively treat and prevent their spread.

6.4.2.2 Non-device-associated infections

Many microorganisms are spread by contact, e.g., MRSA, and *C. difficile* (*C. diff*). These organisms can be spread by touching a person who is colonized or who has an infection (direct contact) or the organism can be spread by touching objects that have the bacteria on them. Bloodborne pathogens such as hepatitis B, hepatitis C, or HIV can be spread in HCFs by contact with an infected person's blood or other body fluids. Simple controls such as environmental cleaning are an important part of the solution. Additional appropriate controls need to be implemented relative to the risk. In highly contagious cases, e.g., airborne infections such as tuberculosis, special negative pressure rooms are needed to prevent the spread of the pathogen.

6.4.2.3 Device-associated infections

It has been estimated that approximately half of all HAIs are device related [10]. Infections caused by devices include:

1. Central Line-Associated Blood Stream Infections (CLABSI),
2. Catheter-Associated Urinary Tract Infections (CAUTI),
3. Ventilator-Associated Pneumonia (VAP), and
4. Surgical Site Infections (SSI).

CAUTI are the most common device-associated HAI.

Microbial biofilms can form on device surfaces and make it easier for an infection to occur. Biofilm is formed when bacteria excrete an extracellular polymer glue-like substance that allows them to adhere to surfaces in moist environments. Biofilms facilitate adhesion and provide a structural matrix that makes them very difficult to break down and remove. Biofilms can be up to 1000 times more resistant to antimicrobial agents than are vegetative microorganisms. Biofilms provide a barrier protecting the complete colony from exposure to cleaning agents as well as antimicrobial agents. Microbes associated with these biofilms are much less susceptible to antibiotics and are difficult to remove from reusable medical devices. In addition, biofilms resist attack and elimination by the host immune system. The biofilm can form from a single bacterial source but often consists of several types of different microorganisms. Biofilm can originate from a patient's skin microflora, exogenous microflora from HCWs, or from contaminated intravenous fluids. Different types of bacteria secrete different polymers with different adhesion properties to attach to surfaces. Bacterial colonization of a medical device can not only impact infection, but it can also affect function of the device. Joint prosthesis has been shown to loosen due to biofilm formation.

Industrial single-use devices

Terminal sterilization is the gold standard for single-use devices. A conservative overkill approach has been extremely effective at minimizing the risk to the patient. Over the past two decades, the CDC has developed one of the most comprehensive data sets tracking HAIs. This has provided insights on the root cause of infection risk to the patient.

The largest signal of inputs that impacts HAIs were due to behavior and procedural contamination of the single-use devices or from challenges to sterilize multiple use devices and not from inadequately sterilized single-use devices. Simple activities such as washing hands as well as more complicated activities such as setting up a sterile operation field and using aseptic techniques during the procedure has had a large impact on reducing infection. It is also noteworthy that the data collection method is sensitive enough to detect increases in infection rates during the recent incident when duodenoscopes were improperly cleaned prior to disinfection or sterilization. On September 26, 2008 the US Government Accountability Office released GAO report number GAO-09-1091R entitled "Health-Care-Associated Infections in Hospitals: Number Associated with Medical Devices Unknown, but Experts Report Provider Practices as a Significant Factor." Per this report the most significant factor affecting the occurrence of HAIs is health-care professionals' improper patient examination and treatment practices. In addition, about half of the 11 experts interviewed for the report cited inadequate preparation of a device for sterilization and improper storage as significant factors in HAIs associated with multiuse medical devices. None of the experts interviewed, nor review of identified relevant articles cited sterilization of single-use devices as a causative factor in HAIs [11].

Most implantable devices are single-use sterile devices and are sterilized by the manufacturer. Implantable medical devices are used to replace a biological structure, support a damaged biological structure, or enhance an existing biological structure. Some implants, e.g., orthopedic plates and screws, are sold as non-sterile and then are subjected to the cleaning and sterilization process at the HCF. An infection can result if the device is not properly cleaned and sterilized before use. Implantable devices should not be reused.

Reusable devices

Reusable medical devices must be cleaned, decontaminated and/or disinfected, or sterilized between uses. It is not possible to disinfect or sterilize a device that has not been properly cleaned first. Cleaning should begin as soon as possible after use. Pre-cleaning should be performed at the point of use. Surgical instrument pre-cleaning should be performed in the OR suite after the patient has left the room or in a pre-cleaning room within the surgical suite.

Manufacturers of reusable medical devices are required to validate at least one cleaning process for the device. Often manufacturers will validate more than one process. Validation is the documented evidence that demonstrates a process will consistently yield product within predetermined specification [12]. The manufacturer will develop cleaning instructions for the HCF staff to follow when cleaning the device based on the cleaning validation.

Surgical site infections

According to the CDC "a SSI is an infection that occurs after surgery in the part of the body where the surgery took place" [13]. At the time of surgery the surgical wound is classified in accordance with an assessment of the degree of contamination of the wound. Wounds are divided into four classes:

1. *Clean.* An uninfected operative site in which there is no inflammation and the respiratory, alimentary, genital, or uninfected urinary tracts are not entered.
2. *Clean contaminated.* Operative wounds that involve entry of the respiratory, alimentary, genital, or urinary tract under controlled conditions and without unusual contamination. There should be no evidence of infection present and a major break in technique should not have occurred.
3. *Contaminated.* These are open, fresh, accidental wounds, and surgeries where major breaks in sterile technique occurred. These might also involve gross spillage from the gastrointestinal tract, incisions in which

acute, non-purulent inflammation is encountered including necrotic tissue without evidence of purulent drainage, e.g., dry gangrene.

4. *Dirty or infected.* Include old traumatic wounds with devitalized tissue and existing clinical infection or perforated viscera. Infection was already present at the time of surgery.

SSIs are further classified by the type of infection that is present.

1. *Superficial incisional.* These infections occur within 30 days after the surgery and involve only skin and subcutaneous tissue.
2. *Deep incisional.* Infection occurs within 30–90 days after the surgical procedures and involves deep soft tissues of the incision, e.g., fascial and muscle layers.
   a. *Organ/space SSIs.* Infection occurs within 30–90 days after the surgical procedure and the infection involves any part of the body deeper than the facial/muscle layers that are opened or manipulated during the surgical procedure.

The impact that an SSI can have is significant. An SSI can increase the patient LOS and can result in a significant impact on the cost of care for the patient. Data suggest that hospitals should expect costs to decrease and revenue to increase as SSIs are reduced [14].

6.5 Preventing HAIs

Many steps can be taken to prevent an HAI from occurring. Improving reporting and surveillance systems will enable the HCF to know if improvement is being made in preventing HAIs. It is important to ensure that the core components for infection control are in place. This includes use of standard precautions, particularly hand hygiene. It is also important to ensure that staff is educated in appropriate infection control practices for the procedures that they perform. Once educated, the staff needs to be held accountable for following correct procedures. In addition, it is important to involve the patients, families, and visitors in using basic infection control practices and in reporting problems.

6.5.1 WHO safe surgery saves lives initiative

"Safe Surgery Saves Lives" is the second global patient safety challenge initiative started by the World Health Organization. The initiative defines a core set of safety standards for surgery to address the problems that complications of surgical care has become a major cause of death, disability, and prolonged illnesses. Avoidable surgical complications account for a large proportion of preventable medical injuries and deaths throughout the world. Adverse events have been estimated to affect 3%–16% of all hospitalized patients and more than half of such events are considered preventable [15–18]. In addition over half of these events occur during surgery [19, 20].

SSI remains one of the most common causes of serious surgical complications. Due to poor systemization, proven measures, e.g., prophylactic use of antibiotics, are used inconsistently. Improving surgical safety is a complex problem that requires numerous steps to implement even basic procedures. As a result of their findings in 2009, WHO created the Safe Surgery Saves Lives campaign. The program consists of 10 essential objectives for safe surgery. One of these objectives is the team that will consistently use methods known to minimize the risk for SSI.

6.5.1.1 CDC SSI guideline 1999

In 1999, CDC first introduced its "Guideline for Surgical Site Infection [21]" Part II of this guideline provided recommendations for the prevention of SSI. This document represented the consensus opinion of the Hospital Infection Control Practices Advisory committee (HICPAC). A new draft guidance on the prevention of SSIs was submitted to the Federal Register on January 29, 2014. Until the new guidance is approved the 1999 version remains in effect. Since the guideline's inception many improvements in infection control practices have been made including: improved operating room ventilation, more effective sterilization methods, increased barriers, better surgical techniques, and increased availability of antimicrobials. Even with these advances SSI remains a significant cause of patient morbidity and mortality, frequently resulting in prolonged hospitalization. SSIs are among the most common HAI accounting for 31% of all HAIs [22]. Approximately 3% of SSIs result in mortality and 75% of SSI-associated deaths are directly attributable to the SSI [23].

6.5.2 Behavior

There are several infection control practices that directly involve the behavior of the people who perform these tasks. Health-care workers must pay close attention to how they perform the following tasks: hand hygiene, isolation precautions, surgical hand scrub, wearing of personal protective attire, and aseptic technique.

6.5.2.1 Isolation precautions

Isolation precautions are used to help stop the spread of germs from one person to another. The goal is to protect patients, their families, visitors, and

HCWs from the spread of infections. Isolation precautions can be divided into two types: standard precautions and transmission-based precautions.

6.5.2.2 Standard precautions

Standard precautions are the minimum infection prevention practice used in the care of all patients all of the time. It can be difficult to tell if someone might have an infection; the infection could be incubating and has not manifested yet or the person might be a carrier who is not affected by the pathogens that inhabit that person's body. Even if a disease is not manifested in a person, it might be possible for that person to infect someone else. Standard precautions are intended to protect people from these unknown situations.

6.5.3 Transmission-based isolation precautions

Transmission-based isolation precautions are an additional type of infection control practice used to prevent the spread of infection from persons who are known or suspected to be infected or colonized with infectious agents. There are three types of transmission-based isolation precautions: contact isolation, droplet isolation, and airborne isolation.

Contact isolation precautions are used to prevent the spread of disease through touching the patient and room surfaces. Droplet isolation is used for patients who are known or suspected to be infected with a microorganism that can be transmitted by droplets. Airborne isolation is used for patients who are known or suspected to be infected with a pathogen that can be transmitted through the air from one person to another.

6.5.3.1 Surgical hand scrub

The objective of a surgical hand scrub is to reduce the release of skin bacteria from the hands of the surgical team for the duration of the procedure [24]. The surgical hand scrub will eliminate transient flora and reduce resident flora. It will also inhibit growth of bacteria on the gloved hand. The Association of Surgical Technologists (AST) and the Association of Perioperative Registered Nurses (AORN) provide guidance on how to appropriately perform the surgical hand scrub. This procedure is performed by the sterile members of the surgical team.

6.5.3.2 Health-care personnel attire

Health-care personnel attire can have an impact on infectious disease transmission. Everyone understands that it is necessary for surgical personnel to wear PPE to protect them from possible exposure to infectious diseases that a surgical patient might have. What is not as well understood is that it is also necessary to protect patients from exposure to infectious diseases from HCWs. This requires that we look at the attire of HCWs in both surgical and nonsurgical settings.

6.5.3.3 Nonsurgical setting attire

Though the role of hospital attire in causing HAIs is not clear, some recommendations have been provided by the Society for Healthcare Epidemiology of America (SHEA) for HCW attire in nonsurgical settings. These recommendations are based on practical, theoretical, and biologically plausible considerations. HCWs should wear short sleeves, i.e., be bare below the elbows (BBE) during patient contact. This includes wearing no jewelry or neck ties below the elbows, e.g., watches, rings, bracelets, etc. If neckties are worn the tie should be secured so that direct patient contact will not occur.

Foot wear should be closed toes with low heels and nonskid soles. Closed toed shoes can prevent blood and other body fluids from contaminating the feet. Shared patient equipment, e.g., stethoscopes should be cleaned between patients. Personal items, e.g., neckties, lanyards, pagers, jewelry, and phones, should be disinfected between patients, and replaced or not used if they become contaminated.

6.5.3.4 Surgical setting attire

Surgical attire should be worn in semi-restricted and restricted areas of the OR. This includes:

- head cover, to prevent shedding of hair, squamous cells, and dandruff,
- facial mask and safety eye wear
- scrub suit,
- warm up jacket, and
- shoe covers.

Head covers should completely cover the hair and be lint free. Facial mask and safety eye wear should always be worn when in restricted areas. A clean scrub suit should be worn each day. The fabric should be low linting, comfortable, breathable and contain shedding of skin cells. The shirt should be tucked into contain skin cells. Shoe covers are used to protect the sterile surgical team members' shoes from contamination from blood, body fluids, and other fluids. These should not be worn outside the OR semi-restricted and restricted areas. In some ORs it is acceptable to wear dedicated shoes instead of shoe covers.

6.5.4 Procedural interventions

(1) Several procedural interventions are used to inhibit the spread of infections in the health-care setting. These include use of antimicrobials, prophylactic antibiotics, surgical clippers, postoperative glucose control, postoperative normothermia, WHO Safe Surgery Saves Lives campaign, and CDCs SSI Guidelines. Each of these interventions is intended to address different aspects of HAI prevention.

(2) There are several ways to prevent microorganisms from being able to move or from encountering a potential host even when the microorganisms are present. Use of PPE can be used to prevent contact with microorganisms. Gloves can be used to prevent picking up organisms on the hands. For respiratory droplets, mucosal surfaces can be protected from having contact with droplets by using masks, goggles, and face shields. Airborne microorganisms can be filtered out of the air with HEPA filters and PPE can be used to prevent contact with these organisms. Common vehicle transmission can be addressed by determining the common vehicle that is causing an infection and then eliminating that vehicle. It is also possible through cleaning, disinfection, and sterilization of medical devices to prevent surgical instruments and endoscopes from becoming common vehicles for transmitting a disease.

(3) Antimicrobials
Antimicrobials are agents that either kill or inhibit the growth of microorganisms. These agents can be classified by the type of microorganism they primarily act against. Antibiotics control bacteria while antifungals control fungi. Antimicrobial chemotherapy uses antimicrobial medicines to treat infection and antimicrobial prophylaxis uses antimicrobial medicines to prevent infection. Use of antimicrobial agents has been common practice for at least 2000 years.

(4) Surgical Clippers
It is generally recommended that hair removal should not be performed prior to surgery. If hair removal is necessary, clippers and not a razor should be used immediately prior to the surgery. The incident of SSI is reduced by using clippers because razors may cause breaks in the skin and a possible pathway for microorganisms to enter the body.

(5) Postoperative Glucose Control
Diabetic patients may need to alter their normal regimen for diabetes treatment when they have surgery. Hypoglycemia increases both in-hospital mortality and the incidence of heart failure in patients

admitted for acute myocardial infarction. Diabetic patients also benefit from close control of glucose levels because it improves the patient's ability to combat infection.

(6) Postoperative Normothermia
Controlling body temperature is a critical element for preventing SSI. The body loses heat during surgery through several mechanisms: radiation from tissues, heat loss through conduction caused by contact with cool surfaces, and convection or exposure to the environment and the temperature of IV. The temperature of the OR is usually kept cool to minimize microbial growth as well as for the comfort of the sterile surgical team members. Hypothermia can result in impaired wound healing, adverse cardiac events, altered drug metabolism, and coagulopathies.

(7) Surgical Asepsis
The surgical team must practice surgical asepsis to prevent an SSI. Surgical asepsis is a set of specific practices and procedures performed under carefully controlled conditions to minimize contamination by pathogens. Although the goal is to maintain sterility, all that one can realistically achieve is to minimize the bioburden that is present. One key concept is the creation of a sterile field that is free of all microorganisms including bacterial spores. The sterile field is maintained by ensuring products and personnel apparel that enters the field is sterile. This is accomplished with sterile drapes including sterilization wraps. Any doubt about the sterility of products/devices being used or personnel must be resolved as quickly as possible; the assumption is that they are unsterile. The surgical team's mantra is "when in doubt, toss it out."

Skin is considered unsterile and must be covered with sterile drapes, gowns, and/or gloves. If anything unsterile (product or persons) contacts a sterile area, then the sterile area is considered contaminated. Sterile items out of sight or below waist level are considered unsterile because if the area is not visible, then it is not possible to ensure that it remains sterile.

In order to maintain the sterile field, it is necessary to ensure that sterile supplies are used, and sterile techniques are observed. The scrub technician or nurse is responsible for maintaining the sterile field and ensuring that proper techniques are used. Basic sterile techniques from sterile gloves being pulled up over the non-sterile gown cuff, handling of sterilized packaging ensuring the contents of the package remain sterile, using aseptic techniques to handle surgical instruments to managing the sterile and non-sterile surgical team must occur seamlessly. Sterile gloves are required to be pulled above the gown cuff. The gown cuff itself is not sterile because it can easily be penetrated and contaminated by body fluids. The contents of the packages must not be contaminated when opened. The exterior of all packages is not sterile; only the contents are sterile following terminal sterilization. Using aseptic techniques when handing supplies and instruments to the surgeon; keeping count of instruments, sponges, and sharps; and monitoring aseptic practice are all important activities. Non-sterile members of the surgical team, including the circulating nurse and the anesthesiologist, must work outside the sterile field and do not wear sterile attire.

6.5.5 Engineering solutions—HCFs

Engineering solutions are effective because they remove the behavioral element which can lapse especially when experiencing time pressures. There are many engineering solutions that can be implemented as part of the design of an HCF that will help to prevent HAIs from occurring. These solutions can include construction design for patient rooms, operating rooms, and procedure rooms; controlling airflow and ventilation; controlling ambient air; controlling traffic patterns and use of protection and barriers.

6.5.5.1 Suite/room design

Surface materials for walls, ceilings, counters, doors, etc., should be chosen for the following characteristics: ease of maintenance, cleanability, seamless construction, and nonporous materials. Ceilings should be at least 10 ft above the floor. Particular attention should be paid to airflow and ventilation.

Airflow and ventilation

Surgical suites, other procedure rooms, and sterile processing areas (preparation and packaging, sterilization, and sterile storage areas) must remain at a positive pressure relative to adjacent areas. This will tend to create an airflow away from these sensitive areas. Special negative pressure rooms used for airborne isolation must remain at a lower pressure relative to adjacent areas and should not have their air changes adjusted when the room is unoccupied. Decontamination rooms should also always be lower pressure compared to adjacent areas.

Certain types of rooms require all air changes per hour to be fresh air, e.g., negative pressure airborne isolation rooms and decontamination rooms. Doors, windows, and doors to pass through machines should be kept closed except when in use. If doors or windows are left open it will be difficult to maintain the appropriate pressure relationships needed for specific types of rooms.

Traffic patterns

Traffic to operating rooms, other procedure rooms, all sterile processing rooms and isolation rooms should be minimized. These areas should have restricted access with all personnel requiring special attire. PPE might also be required in these areas depending on the role of the person working in the area, e.g., sterile surgical team members are required to wear a sterile surgical gown, hat, facial mask, sterile gloves, and shoe covers.

Protection and barriers

Various steps can be taken to protect HCWs and visitors from getting an infection. These include facial masks, eye protection, hoods, caps, shoe covers, gloves, and, for sterile procedures, gowns and drapes.

Facial protection Surgical facial masks serve a dual purpose: they protect the patient from droplet transmission from the surgical team and they protect the surgical team from splash from the patient. When performing procedures where splashing to the face can occur it is also necessary to wear eye protection. Either goggles or face shields can be used for eye protection.

Hoods, caps, and shoe covers Hoods and caps need to completely cover the hair. Their purpose is to prevent hair from falling into a surgical wound during surgery, or on to the dressing during dressing changes or into an instrument set during instrument preparation.

Gloves Sterile gloves must be worn for all surgical and invasive procedures including any vascular access procedure. For surgical and invasive procedures, the glove must cover the gown cuff. In these procedures the sterile glove is intended to prevent the normal flora present on the HCWs hands from contacting the incision or wound. Gloves also serve the dual purpose of protecting the HCW from any infectious organisms that might be present in or on the patient. Double gloving is recommended for most surgical procedures. Non-sterile gloves can be used in isolation procedures.

Gowns and drapes Sterile gowns and drapes must be used in surgery and other invasive procedures. These items have a dual purpose: (1) provide a barrier between the HCW and the patient to reduce microbial and body fluid contamination of the surgical wound and (2) protect the HCW from contact with the patient's blood and body fluids. The entire area of a surgical gown is not considered sterile.

Gowns used as protection should be resistant to blood and body fluid penetration. ANSI/AAMI PB70 describes four levels of protection that a gown could have with Level 1 being the lowest level of protection and Level 4 being the highest level of protection. The level of protection should be chosen according to the volume of fluid expected for the surgical procedure being performed. For nonsurgical and isolation procedures the level of protection chosen should also consider the volume of body fluids expected to be encountered. In all cases, the severity of the contagion also helps to determine the level of PPE required. Highly contagious diseases, e.g., Ebola, require AAMI Level 3 or Level 4 protection. Level 3 is acceptable for visitors who will not have direct contact with the patient. Level 4 protection is needed if there will be direct contact with the patient or their body fluids.

Drapes are used in surgery to protect the patient from contamination from the surgical team and from the patient's own body flora. Only sterile drapes can be used in the sterile field.

Cleaning

Cleaning is an important component of preventing HAIs. This includes both environmental cleaning as well as cleaning the reusable medical devices. There have been cases of patients being infected from a previous patient that occupied the same room [25–28]. Improved surface cleaning and disinfection can reduce the transmission of an HAI. There have also been incidents of patients being infected by improperly cleaned reusable medical devices [29–32].

Cleaning validation Cleaning markers are used to validate a cleaning process. The cleaning marker consists of a medical device inoculated with a clinically relevant test soil that contains various markers, e.g., protein, hemoglobin, carbohydrate, endotoxin, or bioburden. After cleaning, the markers are extracted to measure if the soil has been removed from the device. The manufacturer must determine the acceptance level or concentration of marker that can remain on a device after cleaning. Although there is no current standard for acceptable residual levels that can remain on the medical device after cleaning, AAMI TIR30:2011 [33] provides guidance on the topic. FDA requires the use of a minimum of two markers for validating a cleaning process.

Disinfection Disinfectants are classified as low level, intermediate level (medium level) or high level. The level of disinfection required depends on how the device will be used. Nonmedical devices and environmental surfaces that will contact intact skin only can be low-level disinfected. Noncritical devices that contact intact skin only should be subjected to intermediate-level disinfection. High-level disinfection is appropriate for semi-critical devices. These devices contact intact mucous membranes. Critical medical devices require sterilization.

Chemical and physical disinfectants work by contact; the disinfectant must contact the surface of the medical device for the stated time and at the stated dilution for disinfection to occur. High-level disinfection can also be accomplished with heat. Some washer-disinfector machines provide thermal disinfection.

The efficacy of a chemical or physical disinfectant can be affected by many things. Organic material on a device can prevent the disinfectant from contacting the device surface. The presence of extremely high numbers of microorganisms may require more than the stated time to provide the kill. Different types of microorganisms can have differing resistance to the disinfectant, e.g., bacterial spores will be resistant to all but high-level disinfectants. Devices, such as duodenoscopes, that require high-level disinfection have been associated with a high risk of infection if the item is not adequately cleaned.

Sterilization at the HCF

Medical devices that enter sterile tissue or the vascular system or through which blood flows must be sterile when used. Most reusable medical devices sterilized in HCFs are heat stable and can be sterilized with heat, usually steam sterilization. Some devices require low-temperature sterilization and cannot be sterilized by steam. Low-temperature sterilization processes include: ethylene oxide (EO), hydrogen peroxide gas plasma, vapor-phase hydrogen peroxide, peracetic acid immersion, and hydrogen peroxide/ozone.

Meticulous cleaning of medical devices is required before sterilization. Sterilization processes must be validated by the manufacturer of the device. HCF must follow the sterilization process that was validated by the manufacturer and perform verification each time that the process is run. HCFs should also perform product quality assurance (PQA) testing on all devices sterilized by the HCF. PQA testing involves testing of routinely processed items that represent a product family. It is intended to verify that the process being used by a particular facility for a particular product family is working as specified. PQA testing is used to verify that the device manufacturer's IFU works in the HCF using the cleaning and sterilization equipment available.

Steam under pressure Moist heat under pressure sterilization is the most widely used and the most dependable sterilization process used in HCFs today. This process is nontoxic, inexpensive, rapidly microbicidal, sporicidal and rapidly heats and penetrates fabrics. Moist heat does have some deleterious effects on metal, e.g., corrosion and certain polymers. The goal of moist heat sterilization is to expose all surfaces of a medical device to direct steam at the required temperature and pressure for a specified time. Air can prevent steam from contacting the surface of a medical device. Therefore, it is critical to remove air from the sterilizer chamber for sterilization to occur.

Steam quality and steam purity are also important to the sterilization process. Steam quality is a characteristic of steam reflecting the dryness fraction of the steam and the presence of noncondensable gases in the steam. A steam quality of 0 indicates 100% liquid while a steam quality of 100 indicates 100% steam with no entrained water. Depending on the type of product being sterilized steam quality should be at least 90%–97% [34]. Steam purity is the degree to which steam is free of dissolved and suspended particles, water treatment chemicals, and other contaminants [34]. If steam quality is poor, less than 90%–97% saturated (depending on the product being sterilized), it will be difficult to achieve sterilization temperature on all surfaces of the devices being sterilized. If steam purity is poor, the device may be contaminated by the process and stains may occur on device surfaces.

There are two basic types of steam sterilizers: dynamic air removal and gravity displacement. Dynamic air removal can be accomplished in two ways, by pulling a vacuum or by a process called steam-flush pressure-pulse (SFPP). The equipment differs in how it removes air from the chamber. In gravity displacement, steam is injected into the chamber at the top. As the steam builds up in the chamber it forces the air out through a drain in the bottom of the chamber. This process is slow and inefficient. Device design can result in pockets of air being trapped, preventing steam from contacting all device surfaces. Devices must be positioned correctly in a gravity displacement steam sterilizer. Devices with lumens cannot be sterilized in a gravity displacement steam sterilizer.

In a pre-vacuum steam sterilizer air is removed from the sterilization chamber by using mechanical means to draw a vacuum through the drain at the bottom of the sterilizer. Steam is then injected at the top of the chamber. This process is usually repeated 2–3 times for a total of 3–4 pulses. After the last pulse steam is injected into the chamber and the sterilizer enters the exposure phase of the cycle.

SFPP sterilizers pulse steam into the chamber and use positive pressure to force air out of the drain of the sterilizer. Usually 3–4 steam pulses are used. Once all of the air is removed from the chamber the sterilizer enters the exposure phase of the cycle.

There are two basic types of steam sterilization that are used: terminal sterilization and immediate use steam sterilization (IUSS).

Terminal sterilization It is critical that medical devices are adequately cleaned prior to sterilization. Just like in disinfection, it may not be possible to sterilize a device that is not clean. Devices are terminally sterilized within containers, wrappers, or other primary packaging that is designed to maintain the instruments' sterility and enabling the devices to be stored for later use. At the end of a terminal sterilization cycle, the device must be dry. If a device/instrument set is wet, it is considered contaminated. Terminal sterilization processes are validated to show that they provide a sterility assurance level (SAL) of 10^{-6}. This has been considered the gold standard.

Immediate use steam sterilization IUSS is a method of steam sterilization used on a medical device to be sterilized and used quickly. As the name implies, "immediate use" indicates that the device should be removed quickly from the sterilizer and aseptically transferred to the sterile field. The sterilization cycle used is abbreviated and it is not intended that the device(s) be stored for future use. The same critical processing steps used for terminal sterilization must be followed prior to using IUSS, i.e., cleaning, decontaminating, inspection, and transporting. It is recommended that sterilization containers approved for use in an IUSS process should be used for sterilization and transportation of the devices.

EO sterilization EO is a flammable and explosive colorless gas that is used for sterilization of heat- and moisture-sensitive medical devices. EO is a very effective gas sterilant that has exceptional penetration capabilities. Because of its penetration capabilities, it is necessary to aerate devices sterilized with EO. Aeration is a method of removing residual EO and its by-products from the devices after sterilization. There are several disadvantages associated with EO sterilization.

(1) The sterilization cycle time is lengthy
The cycle includes a sterilization cycle followed by aeration. Depending on the temperature used for sterilization the typical complete cycle time can vary between 10 and 16 h.

(2) EO is also a known carcinogen and mutagen. For this reason, there are strict controls on emission of the EO after completion of the sterilization and aeration processes. In many states abatement and operator permitting is required.

Hydrogen peroxide There are two types of hydrogen peroxide (H_2O_2) sterilization available to HCFs. Vapor-phase H_2O_2 has a rapid cycle time with low temperature. The by-products of the sterilization process are safe and do not require special emission controls or abatement. There is good material compatibility for most medical devices. Some materials like nylon will become brittle and cellulosic materials will absorb the H_2O_2 making validation challenging. A typical vapor-phase H_2O_2 sterilization takes between 55 and 75 min for most medical devices. Penetration of vapor-phase H_2O_2 is not as good as EO, which means that there are some design features such as long narrow lumens that are more challenging to sterilize with this process.

H_2O_2 gas plasma is generated in an enclosed chamber under deep vacuum using radio frequency or microwave energy to excite the gas molecules and produce charged ions. Many of these charged ions are free radicals which interact with essential cell components and disrupt cellular metabolism. The gas plasma cannot penetrate long and narrow lumens and cellulosic materials will absorb the H_2O_2 causing the sterilization process to fail.

Hydrogen peroxide/ozone Hydrogen peroxide/ozone sterilization combines a cycle composed of hydrogen peroxide exposure phase followed with an ozone exposure phase. Ozone can kill both airborne and waterborne microorganisms. It is a powerful oxidant that destroys microorganisms. The highly unstable ozone gas reverts to oxygen and water at the end of the sterilization cycle. There are no toxic by-products to this sterilization method. The process operates at 30–35 °C making it usable for all heat-sensitive medical devices. This process is compatible with a wide range of materials. The hydrogen peroxide/ozone sterilizer can be used for many flexible endoscopes. The manufacturer's information should be checked for any restrictions on lumen size. Ozone sterilization should not be used for products containing the following materials: natural rubber, latex, textile fabrics, copper, brass, bronze, zinc, and nickel.

Peracetic acid Peracetic acid is a liquid chemical sterilant that is a biocidal oxidizer that maintains its efficacy even in the presence of organic soil. The process can be used for high-level disinfection or immediate use sterilization; there is no method for maintaining sterility after the sterilization process is complete. Peracetic acid is used for immediate use sterilization of endoscopes in surgery and for high-level disinfection of gastrointestinal endoscopes.

6.6 Conclusion

The incidence of HAIs is strongly correlated with the activities in HCFs. Terminally sterilized and aseptically processed single-use products have proved effective at limiting this risk as a source of HAI. Although industry still needs to continue to be diligent in its control, the main driver of HAIs is the activities that occur in health-care facilities. Medical device and pharmaceutical manufacturers have the luxury of being able to tightly control incoming materials, environment, equipment, processes, and personnel manufacturing the product. This enables the processes to be highly predictable and repeatable. In contrast, the processes occurring at the HCF are inherently variable and often must be performed quickly. Each patient's microflora, health, and treatment is different. The treatment process as well as the environment is inherently more difficult to control. The net result is that risk to the patient is driven predominately by the more variable processes in the hospital.

In this chapter, we discussed HAIs, what causes them, how medical devices are implicated in them and steps that can be taken to prevent an HAI. Transmission of HAIs is a very complex process that is difficult to control. However, it is important that HCFs take all steps possible to minimize the possibility of an infection to the patient, visitor, or HCW.

References

[1] Antibiotic Resistance Threats in the United States, Center for Disease Control and Prevention, 2013. US Department of Health and Human Services.

[2] WHO, Health care-associated infections FACT SHEET, Downloaded May 14, 2016. www.who.int/gpsc/country_work/gpsc_ccisc_fact_sheet_en.pdf.

[3] Centers for Disease Control and Prevention, Immediate Need for Healthcare Facilities to review Procedures for Cleaning, Disinfecting, and Sterilizing Reusable Medical Devices. Health Alert Network, issued September 11, 2015. Available online at http://emergency.cdc.gov/han/han00382.asp.

[4] CDC/NHSN Surveillance Definition of Healthcare-Associated Infection and Criteria for Specific Types of Infections in the Acute Care Setting, HAI Definitions, January 2013. https://www.cdph.ca.gov/programs/hai/Documents/Slide-Set-20-Infection-Definitions-NHSN-2013.pdf.

[5] HAI Estimates Occurring in US Acute Care Hospitals, HAI data and statistics, CDC, Centers for Disease Control and Prevention, 2011. Available at 222.cdc.gov/hai/surveillance.

[6] Hospital Survey on Patient Safety Culture, User comparative database report, Agency for Healthcare Research and Quality 2016 (2016). page 20.

[7] Background to Clean Care Is Safer Care. WHO. www.whco.int/gpsc/background/en/ Accessed 19 June 2016.

[8] Healthcare-associated Infections (HAI) Progress Report. CDC 2016. www.cdc.gov/hai/sureillance/progress report/ Accessed May 14, 2016.

[9] P. Davey, E. Brown, L. Fenelon, et al., Interventions to improve antibiotic prescribing practices for hospital inpatients, Cochrane Database Syst. Rev. (4) (2005) CD003542.
[10] K. Lillis, Device-associated infections: evidence-based practice remains the best way to decrease HAIs, Infection Control Today (2015). April 11.
[11] GAO-08-1091R Health-Care-Associated Infections in Hospitals, September 26. Available at: http://www.gao.gov/assets/100/95795.pdf, 2008.
[12] ANSI/AAMI/ISO 11139:2006, Sterilization of health care products—Vocabulary, Association for the Advancement of Medical Instrumentation, Arlington, VA, 2006.
[13] FAQS (frequently asked questions) about "Surgical Site Infections," Available on the CDC website at https://www.cdc.gov/HAI/pdfs/ssi/SSI_tagged.pdf Accessed on May 15, 2016.
[14] S. John, W. William, M. Aaron, C. Taylor, F. John, Hadhazy, P. Trish, Final impact of surgical site infections on hospitals. The hospital management perspective, JAMA Surg. 48 (10) (2013) 907–914, https://doi.org/10.1001/jajasurg.2013.2246.
[15] T.A. Brennan, et al., Incidence of adverse events and negligence in hospitalized patients. Results of the Harvard medical practice study I, N. Engl. J. Med. 324 (1991) 370–376.
[16] R.M. Wilson, et al., The quality in Australian health care study, Med. J. Aust. 163 (1995) 458–471.
[17] L.L. Leape, et al., The nature of adverse events in hospitalized patients—Results of the Harvard medical practice study II, N. Engl. J. Med. 324 (1991) 377–384.
[18] United Kingdom Department of Health, An Organization with a Memory, London, 2000.
[19] A.A. Gawande, et al., The incidence and nature of surgical adverse events in Colorado and Utah in 1992, Surgery 126 (1999) 66–75.
[20] A.K. Kable, R.W. Gibbard, A.D. Spigelman, Adverse events in surgical patients in Australia, Int. J. Qual. Health Care 14 (2002) 269–276.
[21] A.J. Mangram, T.C. Horan, M.L. Pearson, L.C. Silver, W.R. Jarvis, et al., Special report guideline for prevention of surgical site infection, Infect. Control Hosp. Epidemiol. 20 (4) (1999) 247–278.
[22] S.S. Magill, et al., Prevalence of healthcare-associated infections in acute care hospitals in Jacksonville, Florida, Infect. Control Hosp. Epidemiol. 33 (3) (2012) 283–291.
[23] S.S. Awad, Adherence to surgical care improvement project measures and postoperative surgical site infections, Surg. Infect. (Larchmt.) 13 (4) (2012) 234–237.
[24] WHO Guidelines on Hand Hygiene in Health Care, First Global Patient Safety Challenge Clean Care is Safer Care, World Health Organization, Geneva, 2009.
[25] S.S. Huang, R. Datta, R. Platt, Risk of acquiring antibiotic-resistant bacteria from prior room occupants, Arch. Intern. Med. 166 (2006) 1945–1961.
[26] M. Drees, D.R. Snydman, C.H. Schmid, et al., Prior environmental contamination increases the risk of acquisition of vancomycin-resistant enterococci, Clin. Infect. Dis. 46 (2008) 678–685.
[27] M.K. Shaughnessy, R.L. Micielli, D.D. DePestel, et al., Evaluation of hospital room assignment and acquisition of Clostridium difficile infection, Infect. Control Hosp. Epidemiol. 32 (2011) 201–206.
[28] S. Nseir, C. Blazejewski, R. Lubret, et al., Risk of acquiring multidrug-resistant gram-negative bacilli from prior room occupants in the intensive care unit, Clin. Microbiol. Infect. 17 (2011) 1201–1208.
[29] A.I. Hartstein, et al., Multiple intensive care unit outbreak of *Acinetobacter calcoaceticus* subspecies antiratus respiratory infection and colonization associated with contaminated, reusable ventilator circuits and resuscitation bags, Am. J. Med. 85 (5) (1988) 624–631.

[30] A. Srinivasan, L.L. Wolfenden, S. Xiaoyan, K. Mackie, et al., An outbreak of *Pseudomonas aeruginosa* infections associated with flexible bronchoscopes, N. Engl. J. Med. 348 (January 6, 2003) 221–227.

[31] Filthy surgical instruments: The hidden threat in America's operating room, in: How Dirty Medical Devices Expose Patients to Infection, February 22, 2012. iWatch News.

[32] Preventable Tragedies: Superbugs and how Ineffective Monitoring of Medical Device Safety Fails Patients. United States Senate, Health, Education, Labor and Pensions Committee, Patty Murray Ranking Member Minority Staff Report, January 13, 2016.

[33] AAMI TIR30:2011, A compendium of processes, materials, test methods, and acceptance criteria for cleaning reusable medical devices, Association for the Advancement of Medical Instrumentation, Arlington, VA, 2006.

[34] ANSI/AAMI ST79:2010 & A1:2010 & A2:2011 & A3:2012 & A4:2013, Comprehensive guide to steam sterilization and sterility assurance in health care facilities, Association for the Advancement of Medical Instrumentation, Arlington, VA, 2013.

CHAPTER 7

Risk to the patient—Quantifying assurance of sterility

Marc L. Speck[a], Harry Frederick Bushar[b], James Niederecker[a], Byron J. Lambert[c]
[a]R&D Quality, Abbott Vascular, Temecula, CA, United States
[b]Retired Statistician, Rockville, MD, United States
[c]Assurance of Sterility Task Force, ASTF, Abbott, Temecula, CA, United States

Contents

This chapter provides a novel look at patient risk by quantifying certain aspects of assurance of sterility related to packaging, aseptic processing, terminal sterilization, and product use at health-care facilities.[a] Terminal sterilization (Chapter 3) with a validated logarithmic reduction in product

[a]Note: reprocessed devices are not included in the analysis of this chapter.

Assurance of Sterility for Sensitive Combination Products and Materials
https://doi.org/10.1016/B978-0-12-805082-8.00007-4

microbial population has served patients well for decades. Decadal studies have not linked terminal sterilization as a contributor to patient infection rates [1–3] except when it was not correctly validated or failed to be executed properly. Aseptic processing (Chapter 4), with terminally sterilized components being manufactured in controlled environments to exclude microbial contamination, is designed for products that cannot be terminally sterilized and has also served the industry well for decades. The use of terminal sterilization with alternate sterility assurance levels (SALs) (for simplification, PNSU★s in this chapter[b]) is another option for products that cannot be terminally sterilized at a PNSU★ of 10^{-6}. Terminal sterilization with SALs $>10^{-6}$ (e.g., 10^{-4}) has recently been expanded upon in the ISO standards (Chapter 9). Packaging as a sterile barrier system or container closure (Chapter 5) is well-established to maintain sterility over the shelf lives of products. The objective of this chapter is to support innovation in sterility assurance to enable patient-centric health-care product innovation (Chapters 2 and 8). This goal is achieved by providing an objective view of patient risk as it relates to health-care facilities (Chapter 6) and the quantifiable aspects of packaging, aseptic processing, and terminal sterilization ISO standards.

A brief introduction to patient risk concepts from ISO 14971:2007 *Medical devices—Application of risk management to medical devices* as applied to sterility assurance is provided in Section 7.1. To make the statistical analysis of this chapter accessible to most readers, a non-statistician's introduction to statistical sampling and confidence bounds as it applies to sterility assurance is provided in Section 7.2. Section 7.3 is a novel statistical analysis of the risk associated with the quantifiable components of standards used[c] in different sectors of the sterility assurance industry including packaging, aseptic processing, and terminal sterilization (a bioburden-based method and an overkill method). For readers not inclined to learn statistics or wade

[b]See Chapter 1, Introduction, for a discussion of the use of the sterility assurance terms across sectors of the sterility assurance field, including sterility assurance level (SAL) and probability of a non-sterile unit (PNSU). As noted in this discussion, different terms are used in different sectors and it is technically inappropriate to use any given term in looking at the quantifiable aspects of sterility assurance across all sectors. Hence, a term PNSU★ is coined for this chapter. PNSU★ denotes the point estimate and confidence estimates of quantifiable aspects of sterility assurance in any given sector.

[c]ISO, PDA, and Pharmacopeia standards apply, especially for aseptic processing; for ease of comparison, quantifiable aspects of ISO standards will be analyzed in this chapter.

through the analysis of the four illustrative cases provided, a good overview of the conclusions is provided in Section 7.3.6.

This risk analysis is put in perspective relative to 'real-world' infection rates (health-care facility infection rates, as seen in Chapter 5) in Section 7.4. Importantly, in none of these four representative analyses does the quantifiable aspect of the respective standard alone provide product sterility assurance; assurance of sterility results from compliance to all aspects of the standard. However, it is helpful to see exactly what the statistically quantifiable aspects of the standards say and do not say about the probability of a non-sterile unit*, PNSU*. This analysis is particularly helpful as alternative SALs are likely to be considered more broadly in the terminal sterilization industry with the publication in 2017 of ISO TS 19930 *Guidance on aspects of a risk-based approach to assuring sterility of terminally sterilized, single-use health-care product that is unable to withstand processing to achieve maximally a sterility assurance level of* 10^{-6} (see Chapter 9). Patient risk acceptability from potential sterility assurance risks are assessed in Section 7.5, and conclusions drawn in Section 7.6.

7.1 Risk concepts applied to sterility assurance

The risk standard ISO14971, *Medical Devices—Application of Risk Management to Medical Devices*, provides an excellent framework to evaluate the risk to the patient. It provides medical device manufacturers with a framework to systematically manage risks to patients, health-care providers (HCP's) and caregivers associated with the use of health-care products. Sterilization deserves special consideration given the potential for harm that could impact, in some cases, large numbers of products or patients. Specifically, the standard describes a process through which the medical device manufacturer can identify and mitigate risks. The key steps in the process are described in Table 7.1.

In Step 1, risk acceptability is a planned activity where acceptable risk levels are defined prior to device design based on desired clinical performance and safety. As per ISO 14971, sterilization risks are deemed acceptable when managed in accordance with standards such as those to be analyzed in this chapter, as given in Table 7.4. In Step 2, risks such as 'inadequate sterilization' are identified along with potential causes. Each risk is analyzed using the risk evaluation criteria to establish its Risk Level. In Step 3,

Table 7.1 Key steps in the ISO 14971 risk management process.

Step	Elements
1. Risk management plan	• Establish risk evaluation and acceptability criteria
2. Risk analysis	• Determine intended use of device • Identify risks • Estimate risk levels using risk evaluation criteria
3. Risk evaluation	• Determine if risks meet acceptance criteria
4. Risk control	• Implement controls where risks do not meet acceptance criteria • Determine if implementation of controls has introduced new risks

risks not meeting the predetermined acceptance criteria are identified so risk controls may be applied, Step 4. Step 4 also includes determination if new risks may result from the use of new controls. This is a key process step as changes to any process have the potential to trigger new risks. Note: see ISO TS19930:2017 provides extensive discussion of factors related to patient risk from infections to consider, in the context of considering a change in the terminal sterilization SAL.

Risk is defined as the combination of the probability of occurrence of harm and the severity of that harm. Risk may be visualized using a two-dimensional risk chart. Various risks for the device are plotted where the occurrence of risks is captured on the *x*-axis and the severity of harm on the *y*-axis. The *y*-axis represents increasing values of severity while the *X*-axis represents increasing values of occurrence. Illustrative risks (*R*1, *R*2, *R*3) are plotted on the chart as shown in Fig. 7.1. *R*1 (1,1) has a low risk since it has a low occurrence rate (1) and a low severity (1). *R*2 (2,2) and *R*3 (3,3) have increasingly high risk.

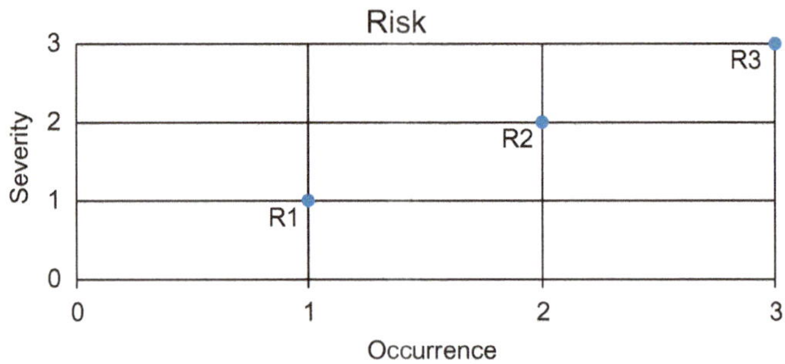

Fig. 7.1 Representative risk graph.

A core concept of ISO 14971 is that medical devices may cause harm if a root cause, which is typically triggered by a sequence of events, occurs and thereby exposes the patient or user to harm. Thus, evaluating risk requires the user to estimate the likelihood of the sequence of events, that is, causes of harm, and the magnitude or seriousness of the harm. Risk mitigation can be achieved in two ways: (1) reduce the probability of the event, for example, sterilization failure, or (2) reduce the severity of the harm. Reducing the harm entails changing the way in which the device fails such that the potential harm is reduced. In the case of a sterilization failure, there is no opportunity to change the potential harm, infection. The focus must be on reducing the likelihood of causes to reach an acceptable risk level. The user can then make decisions on the acceptability of individual risks and the overall residual risk for a medical device.

As manufacturers apply sterilization standards such as those to be used in this chapter (see Table 7.4) and others to control risk, they may discover that achieving a PNSU* of 10^{-6} is detrimental to the device itself based on the materials used in the design. A well-established alternative to the manufacturer is aseptic processing, as discussed in Chapter 4. In addition, a newly clarified option for the manufacturer is the use of an alternative SAL as per ISO TS 19930:2017. This guidance document provides a new regulatory paradigm that frames requisite risk assessment to be completed prior to utilizing alternative SALs in the scenario that terminal sterilization cannot be achieved at an SAL of 10^{-6} (see Chapter 9). Increasing the SAL, for example, providing a 10^{-4} SAL vs a 10^{-6} SAL, for a device can mitigate device performance or safety issues due to the sterilization process, but as would be analyzed in Step 4 increases the risk of infection. Thus, the manufacturer must use the risk management process to assess the higher risk of infection against the patient benefits resulting from the change in sterilization methods.

This discussion related to patient risk will be picked-up again in Section 7.4 after foundational statistical concepts are discussed. Grounding patient risk discussion in the statistics of quantifiable aspects of sterility assurance ensures a focus on the patient and patient risk, as opposed to peripheral issues or legacy paradigms in any given industry sector [4].

7.2 Statistical concepts applied to sterility assurance

Statistical calculations are frequently required to turn data into evidence that supports the safety and efficiency of a process or device. The claim that a process provides a PNSU* below a specified level may be true but regulators ask for statistical evidence. Regulations commonly state that the sampling plans must be statistically valid. In the simplest sense, 'statistically valid' means a conclusion is an accurate representation of the truth. In a stricter and statistically testable sense, 'statistically valid' means the sample sizes can be traced to a predefined statistical objective. This statistical objective is often that the worst-case performance exceeds the minimum value that has been deemed to be acceptable, after accounting for any statistical uncertainty.

This section is aimed at the non-statistician. The level of detail is intended to support the concepts and conclusions without overwhelming the reader. It explains statistics as applied to sterility assurance but does not provide detailed derivations of the statistical concepts or the calculations.

The central statistical concept in this section regards uncertainty. The concept will be introduced using a point estimate and a two-sided confidence interval associated with that point estimate. Intuitive examples are provided to help the reader understand the concepts. The concept of two-sided confidence intervals will be simplified into a single-sided confidence bound. As this chapter is focused on the risk associated with a non-sterile unit, only the upper boundary of the risk is of interest. This is called the upper confidence bound (UCB) of the risk, specifically the UCB of the PNSU*.

After these concepts are developed, point estimates and confidence bounds will be applied to several representative processes that are required to obtain and maintain sterility (see Section 7.3).

7.2.1 Point estimates

The simplest statistical analysis provides the best estimate of the answer. Averages of groups and proportions are examples of this kind of statistical estimate. The value that is calculated is called a point estimate. The point estimate accurately represents the result. If the inference space of the analysis is limited to the data that was used in the calculation, the analysis can stop here. Most often the data that is available is a portion of some larger population, that is, the data is a sample. The intended use of the analysis defines the larger population. Sterilization studies are used to make a statement about the effectiveness of a process that includes manufacturing and sterilization. The data is a sample because the conclusion will be generalized and applied to product built using this process. The population is all product built using the processes and controls that generated the data set.

If the sample that was selected is representative of the population, the sample results are only the most probable result for the larger population. It is possible that the true result for the population is larger or smaller than a point estimate derived from the sample. The single number, the sample point estimate, does not provide any information about how different the population may be. This is illustrated by an intuitive coin flip example.

A coin flipped once may result in a head. It may be accurately stated that 100% of the coin flips (in a sample size of one) resulted in heads. This factually true statement does not provide any information about how likely a head will be in future coin flips. In the technical world, it is appropriate to present data in a format that includes a measure of the uncertainty when it is applied to the population of interest. Answers are usually expressed as a confidence interval or, if the risk is one-sided such as that for sterility, the UCB is reported.

7.2.2 Confidence interval example

Table 7.2 contains 10 columns of 20 randomly generated 0's and 1's. The data could have been generated using a 10-sided die shown in Fig. 7.2. If a nine is rolled a 1 is entered in the table. When any value between a 0 and an 8 is rolled a 0 is entered.

Each entry in the table has a 10% chance of containing a 1 and a 90% chance of containing a 0. In a very large number of rolls, 10% will have a value of 1, as the true proportion of 1's in the population is 10%. Imagine the entries labeled '1' represent a positive sterility test result, a non-sterile unit, while a 0 entry is a negative sterility test result. The expected result is that each column contains 10% 1's, two results out of 20 with the value of 1. In the case of 1's and 0's, an average of the column can be used to represent the count of 1's. In practice, most of the column averages are not 10% (0.1), the expected value. The actual column averages are shown at the bottom of the table. Three of the columns have an average of 0.1. Others columns have an average 0, 0.05, 0.15, and 0.20. These small samples have a large amount of variability. The measured point estimate may not be the true population proportion. The 90% confidence intervals for each column are shown below the average values in the table. To the right of the main table, the grand average of the table is shown along with its 90% confidence interval. These intervals were calculated with the binomial formula.

Table 7.2 Tables of Random values where the probability of the value 1 is 10%.

	Group										
Sample	**1**	**2**	**3**	**4**	**5**	**6**	**7**	**8**	**9**	**10**	
1	0	0	1	0	0	0	0	0	0	0	
2	0	1	0	0	0	0	1	0	0	0	
3	0	0	0	0	0	0	0	0	0	0	
4	1	0	0	0	0	0	0	0	0	1	
5	0	0	0	0	1	0	0	0	0	0	
6	0	0	0	0	0	0	0	0	0	0	
7	0	0	0	0	1	0	0	0	0	0	
8	0	0	0	0	0	0	0	0	0	0	
9	0	0	0	0	0	0	0	0	0	1	
10	0	0	0	0	0	1	0	0	0	0	
11	0	0	0	1	0	1	0	0	0	0	
12	0	0	0	0	0	0	0	0	0	0	
13	0	0	1	0	0	0	0	0	0	0	
14	1	0	0	0	0	0	0	1	0	0	
15	0	0	0	0	0	0	0	0	0	0	
16	0	0	0	0	1	0	0	0	0	0	
17	0	0	0	0	0	0	0	0	0	0	
18	0	0	1	1	1	0	0	1	0	0	**Proportion of the table**
19	0	0	0	0	0	1	0	0	0	0	
20	0	0	0	0	0	0	0	1	0	0	
Proportion	0.10	0.05	0.15	0.10	0.20	0.15	0.05	0.15	0.00	0.10	**0.11**
90% Lower CI	0.042	0.018	0.071	0.042	0.104	0.071	0.018	0.071	0.000	0.042	**0.076**
90% Upper CI	0.283	0.216	0.344	0.283	0.401	0.344	0.216	0.344	0.139	0.283	**0.148**

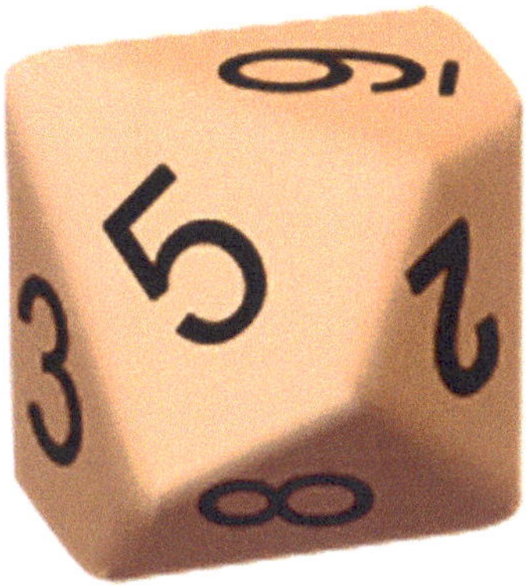

Fig. 7.2 Random mechanism for generating Table 7.2.

Fig. 7.3A shows the point estimates (the proportion of 1's in each of the columns) and the associated confidence intervals that were calculated above. In all, 9 of 10 of the confidence intervals include the true value, 0.1. The intent of the confidence interval is to clearly indicate the region where the truth is likely to fall. The intervals that are shown are 90% intervals. About 90% confidence intervals are expected to contain the true value. In the case of a proportion, the size of the interval is slightly dependent on the value of the point estimate but it is very dependent on the sample size that was used to calculate the proportion. The top data point in the graph shown in black is the grand average for the table. The grand average was calculated using all of the values in the table, 200 data points. It has a confidence interval that is much smaller than the estimates for the groups of 20.

To provide a connection for the reader with the analysis in Section 7.3, this same data is plotted in Fig. 7.3B in the format as forthcoming Figs. 7.4, 7.5, 7.8, and 7.10, using 10^{-9} as an approximation for 0 and a log-based x-axis scale.

Group 9 in Table 7.2 had an average of zero. The die was cast 20 times and a 9 was never rolled. The confidence interval for sample 9 only extends in the positive direction. A proportion is bound between 0 and 1. The upper bound of this confidence interval includes the true value of 0.1. Sample 9 illustrates a very important truth in the context of discussions on PNSU★. It is possible to get a proportion of 0, 0 positive results when the true proportion in the population is nonzero. When the proportion of non-sterile units in the population is very close to 0, as is the desired state for sterility assurance as measured by PNSU★, a 0 proportion in the sample is very likely unless the sample size is extremely large.

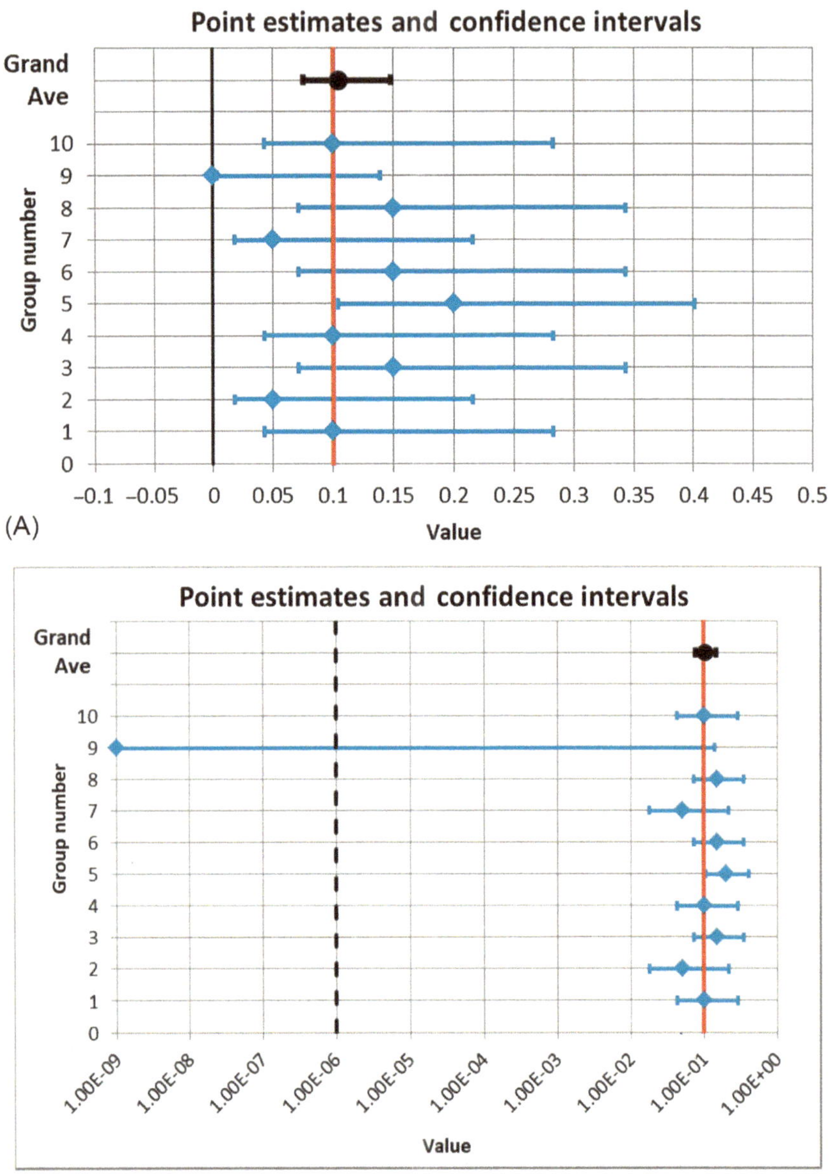

Fig. 7.3 (A) Graphical depiction of point estimates and their confidence intervals. (B) Same data as in (A) using a format consistent with the forthcoming analysis.

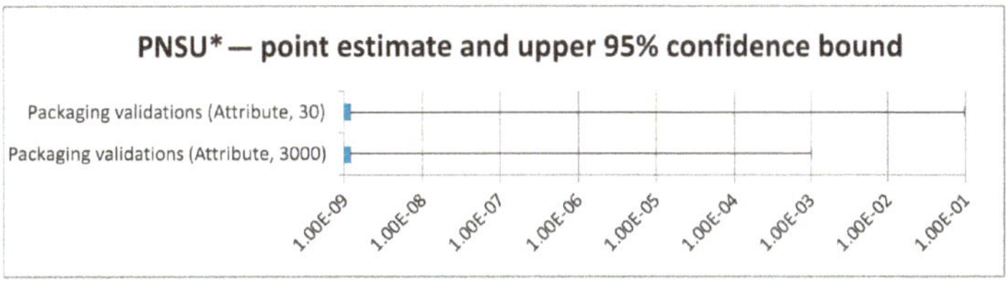

Fig. 7.4 The PNSU* and upper confidence bounds for the packaging example.

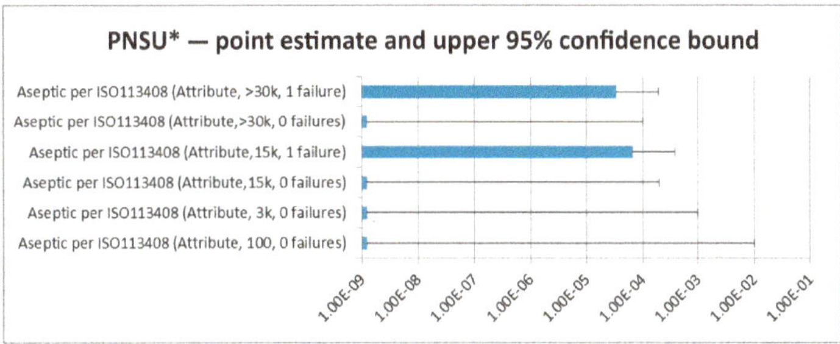

Fig. 7.5 The PNSU* and upper confidence bounds for the aseptic processing examples.

7.2.3 Confidence bounds

The measures associated with the effectiveness of packaging barriers and seals, aseptic processing, and terminal sterilization are single sided. Errors in the estimated results are only consequential in one direction with respect to sterility assurance. An imperfect approximation of the result in one direction creates additional risk while an error in the other direction reduces risk. The upper bound represents the worst possible result from the customer's point of view. The manufacturer desires high confidence and the true result is at least as good as the stated UCB.

In the medical device and pharmaceutical businesses, measures with significant impacts on the health of the patient or the effectiveness of the treatment are typically reported with a high level of confidence. A high level of statistical confidence is traditionally interpreted as a 95% confidence level. The lowest level of confidence that is commonly used is 90%, and this is typically associated with measures that do not have large health impacts and/or significant long-term consequences to the customer.

The grand average of the data in Table 7.2 could be stated as 0.11 (0.076, 0.148). Alternatively, if the risk was associated only with a higher value, the statement could be made that there is 95% confidence that the result is below 0.148. Note: a two-sided 90% confidence interval translates to a one-sided 95% confidence interval.

7.2.4 Statistical analysis types

Before applying point estimates and confidence bounds to assurance of sterility scenarios, one additional foundational concept is helpful. Statistical analysis can be broadly broken up into two types. The simplest analysis is a nonparametric analysis that does not make any assumptions about the underlying statistical distribution and classifies the results as passing or failing against a requirement. This type of data is called attribute data and statistical analysis that is used to evaluate it is nonparametric analysis. The failure or lack of failure of one package and the growth or nongrowth of an aseptic process simulation test, are examples of this type of data. The point estimate of a set of attribute data is a proportion as discussed above.

Parametric analysis is more complex than nonparametric analysis as it is strongly dependent on the identification of the correct underlying statistical distribution. Different distributions are described using different parameters. An analogy to describe the concept of a parameter can be made using geometry. The length of the side of a square is a parameter of a square. If the length of the side of a square is known, everything about the square is known. A rectangle has two parameters. The length of two sides fully describes a rectangle. If the shape is unknown, the correct parameters to describe it are also unknown. The most recognizable statistical parameters describe the normal distribution. A normal distribution is most often parameterized using the mean and the standard deviation. In the parametric analysis, the numeric values in a data set are used to estimate the appropriate parameters for the specific distribution. If the distribution (the shape) and the parameter estimates are known, this information can be used to estimate performance and uncertainty.

7.2.4.1 Nonparametric analysis

The packaging and aseptic processing examples below use nonparametric analysis. A bit of additional introduction is provided here to help the reader get an intuitive understanding of this analysis. Imagine several experiments where dozens, hundreds, and thousands of vials have been aseptically processed and filled with growth media. The expected result for each of these demonstrations is that none (zero) of the vials will show any evidence of microbial contamination. The expected result from the point estimate of all of these data sets is zero, as 0 units with microbial growth divided by the number of units tested as part of the demonstration always equals zero. It should be intuitive that thousands of samples provide more confidence than twenty samples. The point estimate of zero does not depend on how many units were included in the experiment. The numerator in this example is assumed to be zero. While the point estimate is zero in every instance, the worst-case estimate, the UCB of this estimate, is a nonzero positive value. The UCB is very dependent on how many units were included in the sample.

The nonparametric analysis is often used to evaluate the results of the aseptic process validations and for package integrity tests. Sample sizes per batch traditionally do not exceed 10,000 units, and for combination products, the sample sizes can be below 100 units. Table 7.3 shows sample sizes and the associated reliability of the result that can be claimed with high confidence. The table includes three levels of confidence so the reader can see that the conclusions are broadly applicable. With attribute data, hundreds of samples limit the reliability or PNSU* claim to the 10^{-2} level. Thousands of samples raise the level of the PNSU* that can be demonstrated with high confidence to the 10^{-3} level. Demonstrating a PNSU* assurance level of 10^{-4} with high confidence would require nearly 30,000 samples if there was not a single unit with evidence of growth.

One way to understand the UCBs associated with nonparametric sampling is to consider drawing marbles out of an infinitely large bag. It is a given that a certain percentage of the marbles are red; the rest are white. Each draw has the same probability of getting a white or a red marble, as the infinitely large bag has an unlimited supply of marbles. After 22 draws with only white marbles being drawn (zero red marbles), what predictions can be made about the percentage of red marbles? The 90% confidence, 90% reliability location in Table 7.3 (bottom left corner of the table) indicates that 10% of the time 22 draws from the marble bag result in zero red marbles. In other words, if a sample of 22 marbles is taken, and zero red marbles are found, a statistical statement that there is at most 10% red marbles can be made with 90% confidence. Each draw has a 90% chance of a white marble. The chance of drawing two white marbles in a row is 0.9×0.9. The chance of drawing 22 white marbles in a row is 0.9^{22}, or 9.8%. As the percentage of red marbles drops (as PNSU* drops) the chance of drawing many white marbles in a row increases. To make a high confidence statistical statement that the percentage of red marbles is low (the PNSU* is low), a very large number of white marbles in a row needs to be drawn from the bag.

7.2.4.2 Parametric analysis

The terminal sterilization examples below use parametric analysis. A bit of additional introduction is provided here to help the reader get an intuitive understanding of this analysis. The number of microorganisms that are

Table 7.3 The sample sizes associated with reliability claims assuming no failures are observed.

PNSU*		1.E−01	5.E−02	1.E−02	1.E−03	1.E−04	1.E−05	1.E−06
Reliability		90%	95%	99%	99.9%	99.99%	99.999%	99.9999%
Confidence	99%	44	90	459	4603	46,050	460,515	4,605,168
	95%	29	59	299	2995	29,956	299,572	2995,731
	90%	22	45	230	2302	23,025	230,258	2302,584

on/in a product can be treated as an attribute (zero or not-zero) but it can also be treated as a sample from a distribution. Treating data as a sample from a known distribution allows parametric statistical analysis. In this type of analysis, the value (the magnitude) of the result is used in the computation. Parametric data has an advantage in that more information is used from each measurement. Given the same number of measurements, the confidence bound calculated using parametric statistics will be smaller, closer to the point estimate. The weakness of parametric analysis is the reliance on knowing the underlying distribution. If the distribution is identified or selected incorrectly, the results can be very misleading.

7.3 Statistical analysis of risk associated with packaging and sterilization

7.3.1 Introduction to scenarios analyzed

Packaging to maintain sterility, aseptic processing, and terminal sterilization are controlled by a number of international standards, PDA documents, and Pharmacopeia monographs. A partial list of ISO standards to be used for simplicity and consistency in this chapter is shown in Table 7.4. Conformance to these consensus standards facilitates regulatory approvals. The statistical claims associated with the quantifiable components of these procedures will be examined in the sections below.

The analyses of packaging and aseptic processing are based on nonparametric statistics. The use of nonparametric statistical analysis provides a simpler starting point to calculate the point estimate and UCB of the PNSU*.

The analysis of terminal sterilization, a bioburden-based method, and an overkill method are based on parametric statistics and are more complex. The math that is used depends on assumptions about the distribution of microbes and the statistics of half-cycle lethality, respectively. Industry has been challenged to model the distribution of microbes; the Poisson distribution is used despite this shortcoming. Specifically, the Poisson distribution is discrete; its value is defined only for integers (zero microbes, one microbe, etc.); and it requires that the average rate is constant and that each sample is independent of the time or space.

7.3.2 Point estimates and confidence bounds—Packaging

An overview of packaging for terminally sterilized medical devices is covered in detail in Chapter 5. It includes descriptions of test methods that may be used to establish that the packaging is compatible with the device,

Table 7.4 A subset of the standards used in establishing, verifying, and maintaining sterility.

Activity	Standards	Analysis Type	Clause
Packaging	ISO11607-2, Packaging for terminally sterilized medical devices—validation requirements for forming, sealing, and assembly processes	Parametric	7.3.2
Aseptic Processing	ISO113408-1, Aseptic processing of health-care products	Parametric	7.3.3
Terminal Sterilization—Bioburden-based Approach (e.g., Radiation Sterilization, ISO 11137-2:2013, Method 1)	ISO11137-2, Sterilization of health-care products—radiation—Part 2: establishing the sterilization dose	Nonparametric	7.3.4
Terminal Sterilization—Overkill Approach (e.g., ETO Sterilization—ISO 11135:2014 Annex B)	ISO11135, Sterilization of health-care products—Ethylene oxide—Requirements for development, validation and routine control of a sterilization process for medical devices	Nonparametric	7.3.5

allows for sterilization, and prevents microbial contamination. Confidence in maintenance of sterility is achieved from compliance to ISO 11607-1 *Packaging for terminally sterilized medical devices—Part 1: Requirements for materials, sterile barrier systems, and packaging systems* and ISO 11607-2 *Packaging for terminally sterilized medical devices—Part 2: Validation requirements for forming, sealing, and assembly processes.* As summarized in Chapter 5, maintaining sterility is the result of a robust sequential development and validation process. The analysis of this clause focuses on only one portion of the process, quantifiable sample sizes used in package integrity testing.

The methods most commonly used for performance qualification are listed in Table 7.5.

Integrity testing of the package is part of most performance qualifications test plans. This inspection is performed after the packaging system

Table 7.5 Packaging tests most commonly used to for performance qualification.

Purpose	Test	Output	Typical Result
Integrity testing of porous packaging	Visual inspection	Channel dimensions	None found
	Dye penetration	Channel dimensions	None found
	Bubble test	Bubbles/no bubbles	None found
Microbial barrier test methods	Microbial Ingress	Pass/fail	All pass
Seal Strength	Tensile peel	Force	Variable result

has been exposed to mechanical and thermal stresses that might damage the seals. Damage to the seals could compromise the sterile barrier. These inspections are often done using one or more of the methods shown in Table 7.5. While it is possible that some of these methods could generate continuously variable data for statistical analysis, the acceptance criteria and the result are "none," that is, zero defects found in the sample size that was reviewed.

Table 7.3 for nonparametric analysis shows the sample sizes associated with sampling plans where the acceptance criterion is "none found." These are historically common "c equals zero" acceptance sampling plans, where the lower case c is the acceptance number. By definition, the point estimate of zero acceptance number plans is zero. A zero PNSU★, shown as 1×10^{-9} in Fig. 7.4, implies a lower risk than a 1×10^{-6} PNSU★.

Table 7.3 shows that the confidence bounds associated with these point estimates vary with sample size. A performance qualification that required the testing of three batches of 30 results in 90 total samples. Assuming this testing is accepted, the UCB of the PNSU★ would fall in the middle of the 10^{-2} range in Table 7.3. The exact value of the bound is 3.3×10^{-2}. Sample sizes in the tens of thousands would result in an UCB in the 10^{-4} range.

ISO standard 11607-2 does not specify sample sizes or acceptance criterion. It requires three batches and it requires that the sampling (sample sizes) be based on statistically valid rationale. Sample sizes of 30 and 3000 are shown in Fig. 7.4.

The point estimate of PNSU★ for packaging scenarios in Fig. 7.4 is zero (plotted at 10^{-9}) as ISO 11607 requires no defects found. While the sample size of 3000 shown in Fig. 7.4 provides an UCB of 10^{-3}, typical sample sizes result in an UCB higher than 10^{-3}, for example, 10^{-1} for the sample size of 30 shown in Fig. 7.4. In practice, these controls have been successful. Testing extreme numbers of samples to demonstrate a PNSU* of 10^{-6} is not practical or necessary. Confidence in the packaging materials and the maintenance of sterility is not achieved by just performing product integrity testing, as noted at the onset of this clause. Confidence in the seal strength is obtained using parametric methods under worst-case conditions. Receiving inspections at the pouch vendor ensure that the film is consistent. Process controls ensure that the seals are consistent. The packaging validation sample size is just one part of a larger system. It is the entirety of product design control, production controls and the ISO 11607 requirements that ensure that the packaging is fit for its purpose.

7.3.3 Point estimates and confidence bounds—Aseptic processing

ISO 13408-1 *Aseptic processing of health-care products—Part 1: General requirements* and ISO 13408-7 *Aseptic processing of health-care products—Part 7: Alternative processes for medical devices and combination products* provide extensive procedures for controlling the environment and the work practices that are used to manufacture product aseptically. PDA and various Pharmacopeia also have requirements and guidance that are commonly used in the industry. The ISO standard is used in this analysis for consistency with the analysis of the other industry sectors. As summarized in Chapter 4, the assurance of sterility in aseptic processing is based on characterization and control of the manufacturing environment and equipment; personnel training, gowning and general health requirements; and manufacturing aseptic technique. Process simulation requirements are provided to qualify the process, with appropriate tests for sterility. Point estimates and confidence bounds from sample sizes used in process simulations are analyzed in this chapter. Sterility assurance, however, is achieved by adherence to the entirety of the ISO aseptic processing standard. The other portions of the standard are vital to assure sterility but they cannot be analyzed for statistical performance.

The standard makes it clear that the objective is to achieve zero process simulation contaminated units. The procedure also clearly reinforces the importance of investigating any contaminated unit and correcting all root causes.

The relevant information for the statistical calculations is contained in Table 1 of ISO 13408-1:2008. This table has been copied in Table 7.6 and three additional columns have been added when compared to the standard. The number of tests per process simulation was multiplied by the number of

Table 7.6 Process simulations—initial performance qualification information with additional columns.

Minimum number of simulations	Number of Units Tested	Contaminated units in any of the three simulations	Simulation runs affected by contaminated units	Action	Sample sized used in the calculation	Acceptance number used in the calculation	Case # in Table 7.7
3	<5000	w 1	w 1	Investigation, corrective measures, restart validation	300 3000	0 0	6 5
3	5000 to 10,000	1	1	Investigation, consideration of repeat of one process simulation	15,000 15,000	0 1	4 3
		>1	>1	Investigation, corrective measures, restart validation	N/A	N/A	--
3	>10,000	1	1	Investigation	30,003 30,003	0 1	2 1
		>1	>1	Investigation, corrective measures, restart validation	N/A	N/A	--

simulations to obtain the third to last column labeled "Sample size used in the calculation." The acceptance numbers used in the calculations are shown in the second to last column. In certain instances, if a single contaminated unit is found, the procedure does not require a repeat of either a single run or of the entire validation. Calculations for results that meet the letter of the acceptance criteria are shown in this chapter. The values of these two columns are extracted from Table 1 in ISO 13408-1 and provide the basis for the calculation of the point estimate and the UCBs calculated in Table 7.7. The final column of Table 7.6 defines an aseptic processing 'case number' that is used in Table 7.7.

The values for the UCB for each case can be calculated using the binomial formula. In general, underlying math for Table 7.7 is not provided in this chapter. Because the math for Case 6 of Table 7.7 is straightforward, it is provided below for illustrative purposes. The point estimate given in Table 7.7 for Case 6 is zero because the acceptance criterion is 0 out of 300. The upper 95% confidence bound is calculated as follows. The probability distribution function of the binomial equation is given by Eq. (7.1). The sample calculation uses this equation to determine the UCB.

$$P(x) = \left(\frac{n!}{(n-x)! \times x!} \right) \times p^x \times q^{(n-x)} \tag{7.1}$$

where

n = the number of trials (samples).

x = the number of non-sterile units.

p = the probability of non-sterile units for each trial (the PNSU*).

q = the probability of sterile units (must be $1-p$).

and

$P(x)$ = the probability of x non-sterile units, 1—the confidence level.

Table 7.7 Point estimate and 95% upper confidence.

Case	Sample size used in the calculation[a]	Acceptance number used in the calculation	Point estimate of the PNSU*	Upper 95% confidence bound
1	30,003	1	1/30,003 = 3.3 e^{-5}	1.6E−04
2	30,003	0	0/30,003 = 0	1.0E−04
3	15,000	1	1/15,0000 = 6.6 e^{-5}	3.2E−04
4	15,000	0	0/15,000 = 0	2.0E−04
5	3000	0	0/3000 = 0	1.0E−03
6	300	0	0/300 = 0	9.9E−03

[a]The sample size is three times the batch size, for example, for Case 1, 3 × 10,001.

For Case 6, with 300 trials (3 × 100) and an acceptance number of zero, Eq. (7.1) reduces to Eq. (7.2) as x is zero.

$$P(x) = q^n \tag{7.2}$$

Eq. (7.2) can be rearranged as Eq. (7.3).

$$q = e^{\left(\frac{\text{Ln}[P(x)]}{n}\right)} \tag{7.3}$$

Using the data in Case 6 and assuming a 95% level of confidence yields

$$q = e^{(Ln[.05]/300)} = 0.99064$$

PNSU* is the probability of a non-sterile unit (p), and by definition $p = 1 - q$. The UCB of PNSU* = 1 − 0.990064 = 0.009936, 9.9E−03.

If the true value of the PNSU* is 9.9E−03 with a 95% UCB, there is a 5% chance that a test sequence could pass. That is, there is a 5% chance that the result required by the standard, 0 contaminated units in 300 trials, would be observed. In other words, the confidence is 95% that the true value of the PNSU* is <9.9E−03. Referencing back to the marble example, if in truth just under 1% (0.99%) of the marbles in the bag are red, the probability of drawing 300 white marbles in a row is 5%. The confidence is 95% that the true percentage of red marbles is <9.9E−03.

7.3.3.1 Conclusion—Point estimates and confidence bounds—Aseptic processing

The statistical point estimates for the PNSU* when zero contaminated units are found during the testing is zero, show as 10^{-9} in Fig. 7.5. When a single contaminant is found the point estimates are in the 10^{-5} range. The UCB for most of the cases are in the 10^{-4} range, the exception being Case 6 where it was one to two orders of magnitude higher. For Case 6, statistics cannot exclude the possibility that the true PNSU* is in the 10^{-2} range. For the other cases, statistics cannot exclude the possibility that the true PNSU* in the 10^{-4}–10^{-3} range. The sample size is the factor driving these confidence bounds.

In summary, the point estimates and UCB for each of the cases shown in Table 7.7 are shown graphically below in Fig. 7.5.

- For aseptic process simulation tests with zero failures (e.g., Table 7.7, Cases 2 and 4–6), zero out of "n" failures provides a point estimate of zero (shown as 10^{-9} in Fig. 7.5). The UCBs range from only 10^{-4} to 10^{-2}.
- For aseptic process simulation tests with one failure being acceptable followed by retests with no failure (e.g., Table 7.7, Cases 1 and 3), the point estimate is only in the 10^{-5}–10^{-4} range and the upper 95% confidence bound is in the 10^{-4}–10^{-3} range.

As noted at the onset of this clause, it is not the process simulation sample sizes alone that provide confidence in sterility; it is the entirety of ISO 13408 requirements and related process engineering.

7.3.4 Point estimates and confidence bounds—Terminal sterilization; bioburden-based approach

This is a terminal sterilization example of point estimates and confidence bounds from quantifiable aspects of the terminal sterilization validation process. As summarized in Chapter 3, the development, validation, and routine control of a sterilization process start with product definition, that is, defining the product and the microbiological condition of the product. Product manufacturing controls and product bioburden monitoring are required to fulfill this requirement. The sterilization process is then defined to actively reduce the microbial load with the sterilization process in order to achieve the specified SAL (PNSU⋆ in this chapter). This process is then validated; routine controls and monitoring are implemented; product release criteria established and means to maintain process effectiveness implemented. The only part of this process that is involved in the analysis of this clause is a bioburden-based radiation sterilization process definition method, Method 1. The remainder of the standard cannot be statistically analyzed but is the entirety of what assures sterility.

The previous two examples are based on nonparametric statistical analysis. The following two Terminal Sterilization examples are based on parametric analysis, where the analysis is based on an assumed underlying distribution. In each example, the Method is broken down into two parts, Parts A and B, and statistics are defined for each part to make the analysis more understandable. Only a relatively small portion of the underlying mathematics is included to give the reader a sense of the math but to allow the flow of the chapter to progress without interruption.

The specific method used in this clause is a radiation sterilization bioburden-based Method, Method 1, from ISO 11137-2:2013 *Sterilization of health-care products—Radiation—Part 2: Establishing the sterilization dose.* It is for a product with an assumed true average bioburden of 3.5 to provide an example of the confidence bounds for a bioburden-based validation method. An assumed average bioburden of 3.5 has been chosen because the low value highlights concepts of the statistical analysis in this scenario, that is, differentiation of doses selected from Table 5 of Method 1. This Method provides a path to establish an acceptable radiation dose to generate a targeted PNSU⋆. A schematic representation of the procedure described in Method 1 is provided below in Fig. 7.6.

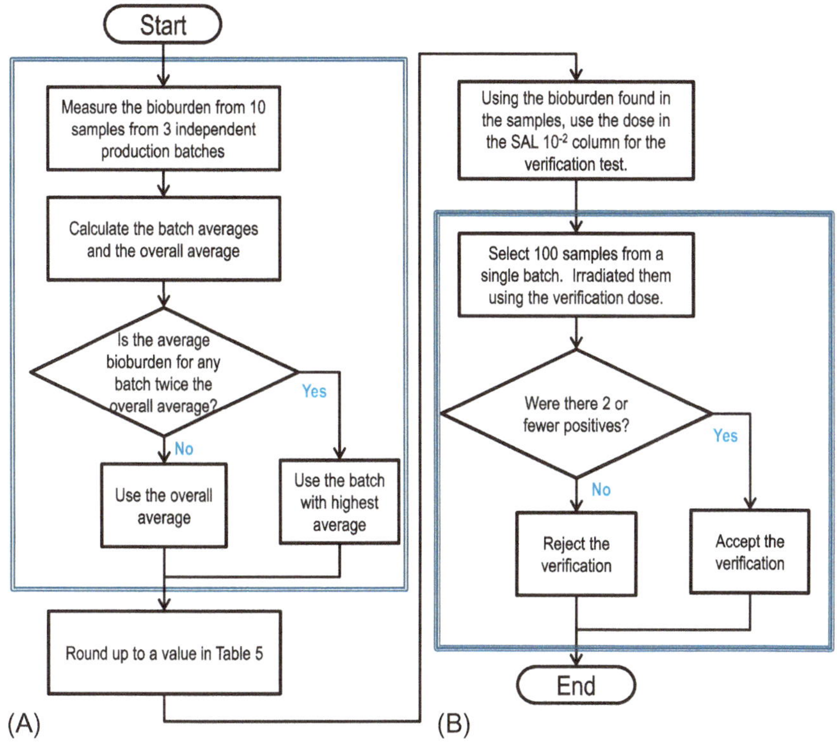

Fig. 7.6 A schematic flowchart of Method 1 per ISO 11137-2.

7.3.4.1 Section A

Section A shown in Fig. 7.6 highlights the steps that are used to establish the level of bioburden in the product. The ideal statistical situation is complete homogeneity of lots and samples within a lot. Using these simplified assumptions, statistics will be used to obtain approximate confidence boundaries for the level of bioburden. This is the first part of the parametric statistical analysis required to obtain the overall point estimate and confidence bound for this example.

It is important to note that in this scenario the bioburden value of 3.5 and the associated Poisson distribution of bioburden values have been selected to illustrate statistical calculations of the relation between bioburden variability and quantitative analysis of PNSU*. Real-world bioburden variability can be significantly greater as seen by the standard's accommodation of batches with bioburden average being twice that of the overall average of three batches as shown in Part A above. Conclusions remain instructive.

As noted above (see Section 7.3.1), the distribution of microbes is assumed to be described by the Poisson distribution. Approximate confidence intervals for Poisson distributions are provided by Eq. (7.4). The lower confidence bound (LCB) is used as the illustrative worst-case scenario in this analysis and z-alpha is the quantile of a normal distribution evaluated at the defined alpha level, lambda is the mean of the Poisson process and n is the number of samples used to establish the mean. Alpha represents the percent of the samples when this result is expected to occur.

$$LCB = Z_{\alpha} \times \sqrt{\lambda / n} \tag{7.4}$$

Table 7.8 shows the probability of getting various bioburden results in 30 samples based on the Poisson distribution assumption. Consider that there is a very large batch of samples and the true bioburden has an average of 3.5. If hundreds of groups of 30 samples are tested, the average of each group will be a bit different. Table 7.8 uses Eq. (7.4) to determine that 0.1% of the sample will have an average of 2.4. When the standard is followed, this would round to 2.5. The table also shows that 7% of the time the average will be below 3 (2.996 in the table) will be used. This is important as a 95% confidence bound is typically used for risks that have a large impact on patient safety. The 95% confidence bound of this sampling plan does not result in selecting the true bioburden level of 3.5 from Table 5 of ISO 11137-2:2013 in this situation.

It should be noted that 91% of the time an average of 3.5 or greater will be used. In addition, a bioburden average of >3.5 will occur 50% of the time (3.5 is the mean value). This is a consequence of the standard indicating to use the 'next greater value' in Table 5 of ISO 11137-2:2013.

The statistical conclusion after reviewing the portion of the procedure labeled Section A in Fig. 7.6 is if the procedure in the standard is followed, approximately 7% of the time a bioburden level of 3 or lower will be used,

Table 7.8 The probability of various average results from 30 samples where the true average is 3.5.

alpha	*Z* alpha	LCB	Result
0.1%	**−3.090**	**1.056**	**2.444**
1.0%	−2.326	0.795	2.705
5.0%	−1.645	0.562	2.938
7.0%	**−1.476**	**0.504**	**2.996**
8.0%	−1.405	0.480	3.020
10.0%	−1.282	0.438	3.062

and 50% of the time a bioburden level of 4 or higher will be used, to identify the radiation dose for the verification run when the true level is 3.5.

7.3.4.2 Section B

The analysis in Section A established that a sampling error might result in misidentifying the average bioburden a modest fraction of the time for bioburden estimates below the average value and 50% of the time for bioburden estimates above the average. Section B will provide illustrative statistical analysis for the underestimate of bioburden.

For Method 1, the verification testing is intended to demonstrate the selected level of radiation will result in a 10^{-2} PNSU★. This demonstration supports the identification of a radiation dose designed to achieve a selected PNSU★, most often a 10^{-6} PNSU★. The next step of the analysis related to the ISO 11137-2 components shown in Section B (Fig. 7.6) will use operational characteristic curves (OCC or OC curves) to determine if the verification tests prescribed in the standard would detect the error in the estimate of the bioburden level.

OC curves graphically illustrate the ability of a sampling plan to discriminate between acceptable and unacceptable results. The OC curve in Fig. 7.7 will be used to introduce the concepts of acceptance sampling and OC curves. It is not the OC curve for the plan described by the standard. The curve shown in Fig. 7.7 describes the performance of a sampling plan where 299 samples ($n=299$) are tested and none are allowed to fail ($c=0$). The x-axis of the curve is the fraction defective in the batch. The y-axis is the probability of passing the sampling plan given the fraction defective on

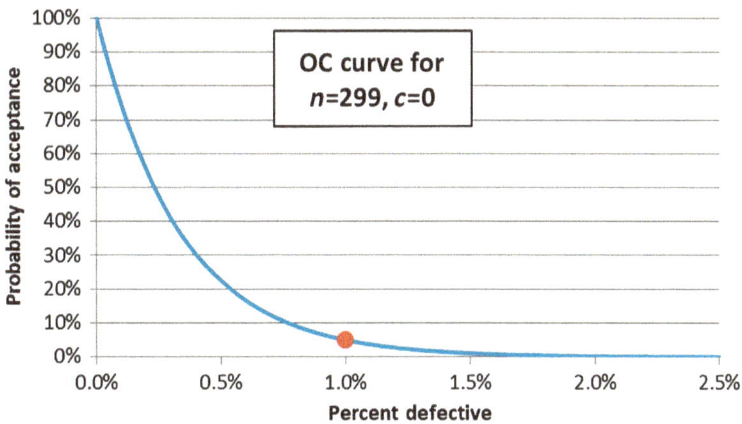

Fig. 7.7 A general OC curve.

the *x*-axis. At 1% defective, the probability of acceptance is 5%. This value is shown with a red dot. The probability of detection (1 minus the probability of acceptance) is 95%. This plan provides a 95% confidence of detecting a batch that is 1% defective or worse. Non-sterile samples can be considered defective. Note that passing this plan every time, having a high probability of acceptance, requires a very low fraction defective.

The Method 1 verification test in Section B (Fig. 7.6) is a sampling plan. 100 samples are taken, processed such that the expected probability that any unit contains a microorganism is one in a hundred, or has a PNSU* of 10^{-2}. The OC Curve for the verification plan identified in Method 1 is shown in Fig. 7.8. The *x*-axis has been modified slightly. The scale has the same unit of measure, percent defective, but it uses a log scale that is more appropriate for sterilization defect levels. The concept of the OC curve is relevant to this verification testing as each sample is either sterile or non-sterile. The targeted fraction defective, the PNSU*, is 1 in 100 units or fewer, or $1E^{-2}$. This location is shown on the OC curve with a green line. This line intersects the OC curve at 91%. If the PNSU* of the batch is exactly as planned, the verification testing will fail 9% of the time. A red line is shown where the OC curve has a probability of acceptance of 5%. This verification plan provides 95% confidence that the sterilization level is $6E^{-2}$.

On average Section A (Fig. 7.6) will overestimate the level of bioburden with the round-up rule. About 50% of the time the result of the sample in Section A will be 3.5 or higher. As per the standard, this value would be rounded up. This increases the radiation dose that is used in verification testing <u>and</u> in the final process. About 7% of the time the bioburden level will

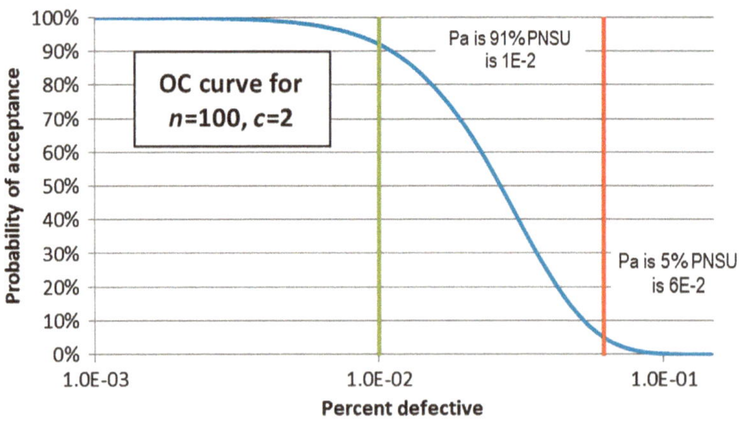

Fig. 7.8 OC curve for the sampling plan described in the standard.

be underestimated. This underestimation will result in the use of a lower radiation level as part of the verification testing and in the final processes. The OC curve shown in Fig. 7.8 demonstrates that the verification testing step cannot be expected to detect this 7% underestimation with high confidence.

This simplified analysis using the low bioburden average of 3.5 CFU that for some levels of bioburden the UCB of the PNSU⋆ is $>1\times10^{-6}$.

7.3.4.3 Conclusion—Point estimates and confidence bounds—Terminal sterilization; bioburden-based approach

The PNSU⋆ provided by ISO 11137-2:2013 Method 1 is dependent on the level of bioburden. In some cases, the procedure used to estimate the level of bioburden will result in a result lower than the truth. The verification component of the standard is not likely to detect this underestimate. While the UCB is in the 10^{-6} range, this quantifiable aspect of the standard does not universally result in providing the targeted PNSU⋆ (typically $<1\times10^{-6}$) with high confidence, although it is close. This result is illustrated in Fig. 7.9. It is noted again that it is compliance with the entirety of the standard that assures sterility, not merely the bioburden estimates and verification dose levels.

7.3.5 Point estimates and confidence bounds—Terminal sterilization; overkill method

This is another terminal sterilization example of point estimates and confidence bounds from quantifiable aspects of the terminal sterilization validation process. As noted in Section 7.3.4, there are many aspects of the terminal sterilization process in ISO standards to assure sterility. This is only part of the standards' procedures; it is the quantifiable part of the ethylene oxide process definition Overkill Method. The remainder of the standard cannot be statistically quantified but is the entirety of what assures sterility.

EO sterilization, ISO 11135:2014 *Sterilization of health-care products—Ethylene oxide—Requirements for development, validation and routine control of*

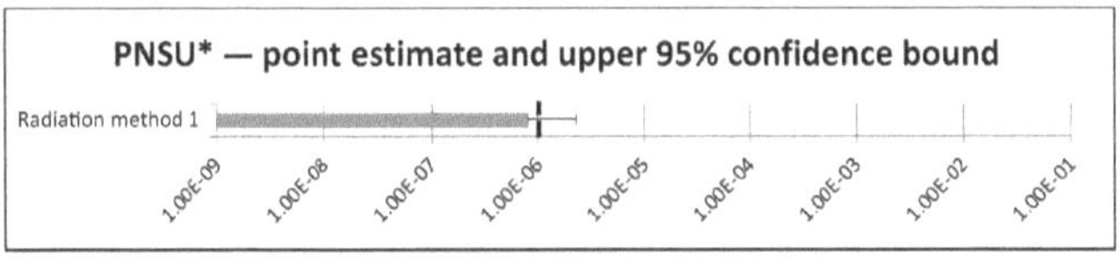

Fig. 7.9 The PNSU* and upper confidence bounds for the ISO 11137-2 Method One.

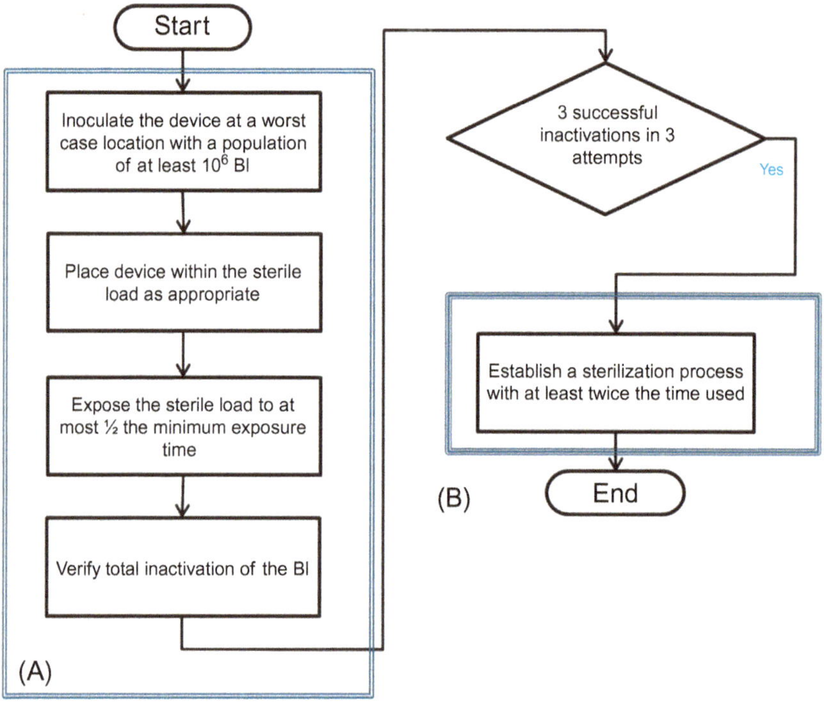

Fig. 7.10 A schematic flowchart of the steps described in ISO11135 Annex B.

a sterilization process for medical devices, Annex B, provides an example of an overkill method. It describes a procedure that can be used to verify that an ethylene oxide sterilization cycle achieves a 12 log reduction of active bioburden and a PNSU* $<10^{-6}$. The procedure described in the half-cycle approach is summarized in Fig. 7.10. The steps and rules contained in this standard will be used for the final illustration of point estimates and confidence bounds.

7.3.5.1 Section A

Section A of Fig. 7.10 includes the steps that demonstrate that a sterilization cycle that is one-half of the planned duration results in complete inactivation of, for example, one million microbes on the biological indicator. No viable microbes may be recovered in any of the required three consecutive demonstrations. The point estimate of the recovered population is zero. The upper 95% confidence bound of the microbial distribution will be shown to be <1 microbe out of one million initial microbes.

The number of recovered microbes is a sample from a Poisson distribution (Eq. 7.4). A single parameter lambda fully describes the distribution. The value of lambda is also the average value of the Poisson distribution. Assuming the true average number of microbes per unit after a half-cycle is one (lambda is one), the probability of getting a zero result in a single sample can be calculated using the Probability Mass Function (PMF) for the Poisson distribution shown in Eq. (7.5). Given a k of zero (zero microbes), the equation reduces to 1 over *e*. There is a 36.788% of a value of zero on any sample.

$$P_k = \frac{\lambda^k \times e^{-\lambda}}{k!} \tag{7.5}$$

where

k is the number of observations.

P_k is the probability of k observations.

Basic probability theory states the probability of getting a zero twice in two attempts is $P_k \times P_k$. The probability of getting zero 3 times in a row is 0.367888 cubed or 4.98%. There is less than a 5% chance of getting three zero values in three consecutive attempts if the true value of lambda is as large as one. The upper 95% confidence bound of this estimate is the average (λ) is <1.

The spore-log-reduction (SLR) for the fraction negative results are defined in Eq. (7.6). The log of the final population is required to be zero. The log of zero is undefined and the standard states that the SLR can be reported as ">log N_0" if one is used for N_U, the final population.

$$\text{SLR} = \log N_0 - \log N_U \tag{7.6}$$

where

N_0 is the initial population,

N_U is the final population.

Using one for the value of N_U is conservative as the upper 95% confidence bound for lambda is <1. The analysis above supports that the 95% confidence for the average value of N_U is <1.

The required initial bioburden load of one million spores and the required final result of one are substituted into Eq. (7.6). The result is a spore log reduction of 6. There is 95% confidence that the spore log reduction is demonstrated in Section A is at least 6.

7.3.5.2 Section B

The definition of D-value requires that if ETO exposure time is doubled, the SLR also doubles from 6 to 12. The standard requires at least doubling the exposure time. The overkill approach provides 95% confidence of a 12 log reduction in the bioburden.

7.3.5.3 Conclusion—Point estimates and confidence bounds—Terminal sterilization; overkill method

The point estimate for the PNSU* for the Overkill method is zero (shown as 10^{-9} in Fig. 7.11) and the UCB is 1×10^{-6}, one part in a million. This method provides a high confidence demonstration that the PNSU* is $<1\times10^{-6}$. The point estimate and the UCB are illustrated in Fig. 7.11. It is important to note that while the UCB of this terminal sterilization method demonstrates a PNSU* of $<10^{-6}$, it is still in compliance with the entirety of the standard that assures sterility.

7.3.6 Summary of statistical analysis

The quantifiable aspects of standards that are intended to ensure medical devices, as used by the customer, have a low probability of being non-sterile were reviewed from a statistical point of view. This analysis is not an exhaustive review of the standards, it was a survey. Most of the testing used to demonstrate acceptability as per the standards results in pass/fail data. This data is analyzed using nonparametric statistics and is shown in Fig. 7.12 in blue. Two of the methods provide data that can be analyzed using parametric statistics. These are shown in green in the graph. Fig. 7.12 compiles the data previously reported in Figs. 7.4, 7.5, 7.9, and 7.11.

The UCBs that would result from following the quantifiable aspects of the standards were calculated. Most of the standards that were examined require the point estimate of the PNSU* to be $<1\times10^{-6}$. Only a single standard that was included in the analysis, for terminal sterilization using the overkill method, demonstrated an UCB with a PNSU* at this level. The bioburden-based terminal sterilization method was close to this range. The statistical UCB of PNSU* that is demonstrated as per packaging and aseptic processing standards is typically much greater, that is, 10^{-4} or greater. As a group, the quantifiable aspects alone called out in the standards do not provide statistical evidence that the associated PNSU* is $<1\times10^{-6}$.

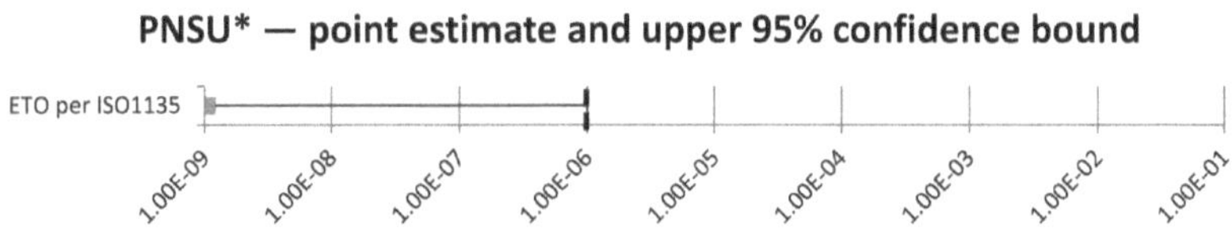

Fig. 7.11 The PNSU* and upper confidence bounds for the ISO 11135:2014, Annex B.

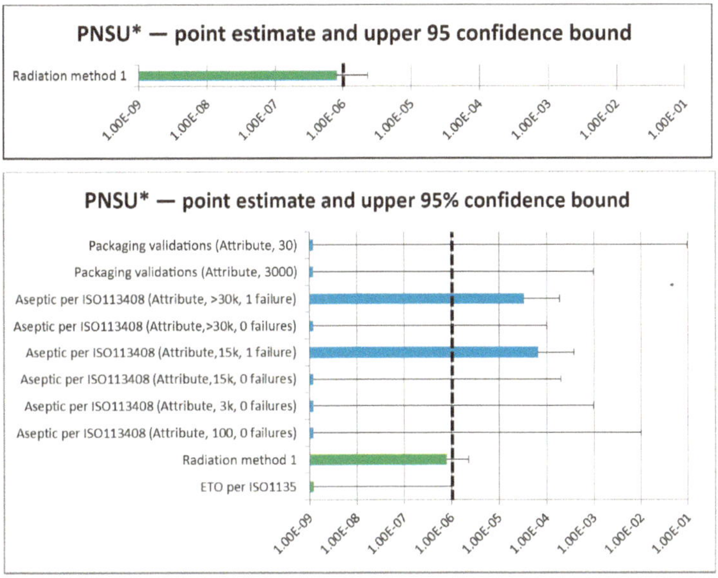

Fig. 7.12 The point estimates and the upper confidence bounds of select scenarios.

The lack of strong statistical evidence provided by the quantifiable testing of the standards is not a statement that these standards are lax. Final overall system testing is a single part of the design control effort that ensures the product is free from pathogens. Using packaging as an example, the selection and testing of the barrier materials, the development and control of sealing methods, the testing of the seal strength, the use of very challenging test conditions on the completed package, and control of the distribution chain all contribute to ensure that the packaging is robust and up to the challenge of maintaining sterility. The protection that these steps provide cannot be easily included in the statistical calculations focused on the as-shipped configuration.

Some methods, because they can be modeled parametrically, provide a practical pathway to demonstrating a very low PNSU* with high confidence. With other methods, aseptic processing, for example, the final process can only be tested nonparametrically. This reality precludes any practical demonstration of very low PNSU* levels with high confidence for the overall process. The standards acknowledge this limitation and the acceptability of this limitation in order to provide a sterile product to meet the needs of patients. The ISO 13408-7 standard also recognizes that active reduction of bioburden in terminal sterilization is preferred over the exclusion of bioburden in aseptic processing. However, in order to meet patient needs, aseptic processing is acceptable and has served patients well for decades.

The discussion below related to patient risk picks-up from clause 7.1. The intervening discussion of the statistics of quantifiable aspects of sterility assurance grounds the following patient risk discussion and ensures a focus on the patient and patient risk, as opposed to peripheral or nonvalue-added sterility-related issues or paradigms in any given industry sector.

7.4 Relative patient risks from various industry sectors compared to real-world infection rates

Estimating the risk of infection for a sterile device will entail considering the sources of harm (failure modes) and their likelihood of impacting the overall risk in the system. There are multiple factors that could be viewed individually or as a sequence of events which can influence the likelihood of infection as shown in Fig. 7.13. Each factor has a potential likelihood of occurrence, with all factors resulting in a collective or total likelihood of occurrence.

7.4.1 Estimates of infection probabilities

Estimates of infection probabilities will be assigned for a hypothetical terminally sterilized product with a process to achieve a PNSU⋆ of 10^{-6}, the P1 estimate. Even with conservative assumptions, when the estimates of infection probabilities are assessed, the PNSU⋆ is seen to be significantly less, for example, 10^{-7} or 10^{-8}.

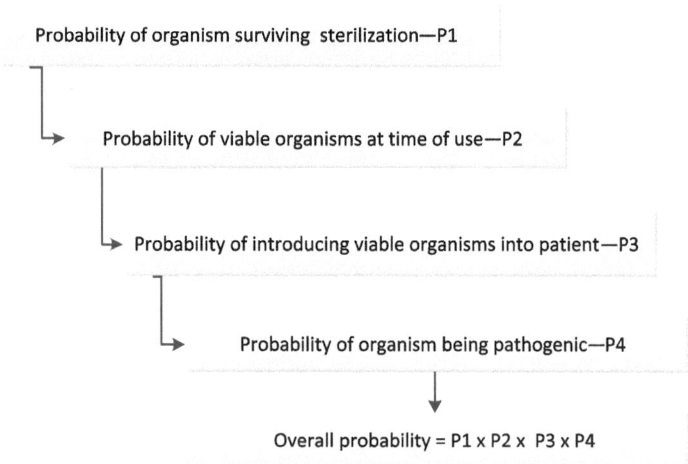

Fig. 7.13 Infection risk factors.

In light of new regulatory paradigms in ISO TS19930:2017 as described in Chapter 9, this example could have used a hypothetical terminally sterilized product with a process to achieve a PNSU* of 10^{-4}, the P1 estimate, resulting in a real-world estimate of a PNSU* of 10^{-5} or 10^{-6} as shown below. The analysis could also have used a hypothetical aseptic process with a P1 estimate from Table 7.7. Estimates of P2, P3, and P4 will be similar for all of these scenarios.

7.4.1.1 Probability of P1

The basic probability of an organism present on a sterile product is initially estimated via the PNSU* for terminal sterilization processes and by the estimate of contamination rate in aseptic processing (quantified in Section 7.3.3 as the UCB of the aseptic process).

Terminal sterilization processes result in SAL ranges. For example, a radiation sterilization dose range of 20–35 kGy that would provide a PNSU* range of 10^{-6} to 10^{-9} or less, as discussed below and seen in Fig. 7.14. However, for a risk analysis, the lowest assurance of sterility must be assumed, which would be 10^{-6} for this particular PNSU* range. For purposes of this analysis, a standard assurance of sterility, PNSU* of 10^{-6}, is assumed. Hence $P1 = 1 \times 10^{-6}$.

7.4.1.2 Probability of P2

The next factor in this analysis is the probability of viable organisms at time of use. This factor is contingent on several factors including the storage environment, the time of storage, types of organisms and their ability to survive.

In the manufacture of health-care products, the environmental organisms are usually expected to be similar, regardless of the nature of the product [5]. The environmental isolates recovered during the manufacture of biologics and tissue-based products are typically the same types as those recovered in medical device manufacturing. Because the manufacture of biologics and tissue-based products relies heavily on screening of materials and high-level disinfection, the resulting bioburden of both categories of health-care products is, in most cases, made up of commonly encountered microorganisms from activities related to the environment and handling. Any significant difference between the bioburden of these two categories of health-care products will usually be due to the bioburden found on the raw materials.

This common spectrum of bioburden flora is the basis of the effectiveness of most terminal sterilization processes. Therefore, although the

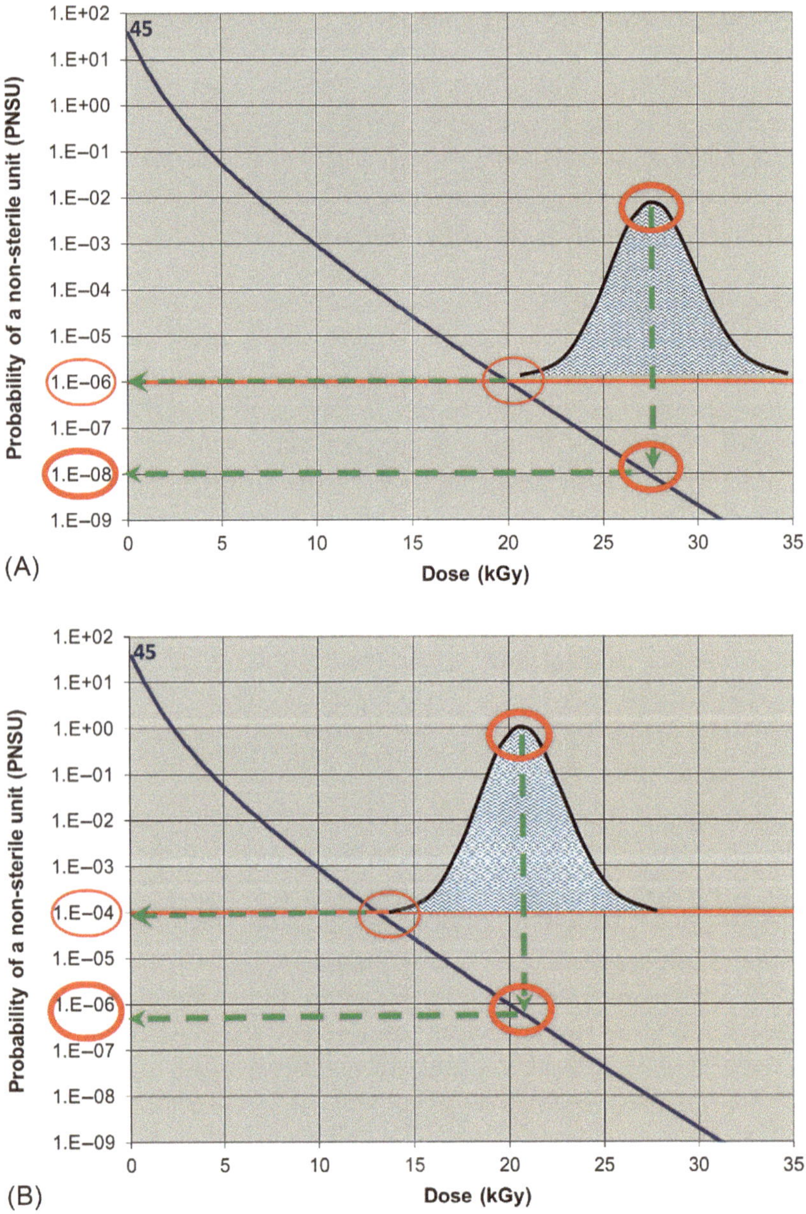

Fig. 7.14 (A) Radiation sterilization dose-response curve—SAL 10^{-6}. (B) Radiation sterilization dose-response curve—SAL 10^{-4}.

expectation of a survivor of a sterilization process is extremely low, there is also the expectation that any survivor should also be one that is resistant to the particular sterilization process. In that case, it should be relatively easy to research the general ability of an organism that might survive the sterilization process to survive the storage environment (temperature and humidity) as well as the time of storage.

On a product that does not support microbial growth, it is well understood that bioburden dies off with the passage of time [5]. Additionally, small numbers of organisms on a device may be of little consequence to the patient; however, the ability of the organisms to multiply is key to this analysis. Bacterial and fungal growth requires consumables (nutrients) and the right environment, that is, temperature and pH. Fortunately, nutrients are generally unavailable on most sterile devices. Microorganisms have an absolute requirement for water and water availability has a profound effect on survival and growth [5]. The presence of water or moisture may be present in some packaging or devices; however, this is not the norm. Some organisms can grow in the absence of air (anaerobic), however, most require oxygen (aerobic). Thus devices packaged in an inert gas limit microbial growth. There is an optimum pH over which microorganisms can grow. Bacteria grow best around pH 7 but many molds can tolerate more acidic conditions, pH 5–6. Some microorganisms are surprisingly tolerant of hostile pH environments [5]. The typical environment for a sterile device is pH neutral and does not deter growth. As with pH, there is an optimum temperature range for microbial growth. Low-temperatures slow growth rates while higher temperatures increase growth rates. Storage environments are varied and may include hot or cold temperatures and dry or moist conditions for periods of time during shipping. Typical hospital device storage is at room temperature which does not deter growth.

Knowing the length of time and storage/transport conditions that would occur between sterilization and patient use, one can estimate the probability of survival. Another factor is the possibility that the organism was damaged from the sterilization process. All of this information can be used to estimate the probability of an organism that might have survived sterilization to still be viable at the time of use of the product.

A conservative example of a value for P2 would be a 1 in 2 chance that an organism would still be viable at the time of use, possibly based on the bioburden having spores, the product being one that may support growth, the lead time between sterilization and use being shorter, and there being controlled shipping/storage conditions. A more realistic example of a value for P2 would be a 1 in 10 chance that an organism would be viable at the time of use on a patient, possibly based on the bioburden having vegetative bacteria only, the product being one that does not support growth, the lead time from sterilization to use being longer, and there being uncontrolled/hostile shipping/storage conditions.

If a product is capable of supporting growth, then maybe a 1 in 1 likelihood of a surviving organism still being viable at the time of use, and at minimum P2 = 1.

For this example P2 (conservative case) = 1 while P2 (more aggressive case) = 0.1 (1×10^{-1}).

7.4.1.3 Probability of P3

The third factor is the probability of introducing viable organisms into the patient. This factor assumes the surviving organism (a) is transferred from the package to the device if it is on the interior of the package, (b) is resident on the device, (c) is not removed during device preparation, (d) resides on a part of the device that contacts the patient, or (e) resides on a part of the device that contacts the user and is transferred to the patient and the organism is not removed during handling. Using facts such as the portion of the device that contacts the patient being 20% of the device, one could use a conservative likelihood of 1 in 5. In this example P3 = 0.2 (2×10^{-1}.) A very conservative approach would assume the organism is introduced despite the location, possibility of removal or possibility of transfer.

For this example P3 (conservative case) = 1 while P3 (more aggressive case) = 0.2 (2×10^{-1}).

7.4.1.4 Probability of P4

The fourth factor, the probability of an organism being pathogenic is contingent on the types of organisms prevalent in the manufacturing environment and on the bioburden of the product materials. Organisms from the manufacturing environment are of less concern since there is no direct product contact, however, controls are still required. Environmental contamination of dry surfaces such as floors and walls comprise mainly Gram-positive rods, cocci, and fungal spores. Gram-negative bacteria are more susceptible to the lethal effects of drying, but small numbers may persist on dry surfaces for substantial periods [6].

Contamination from process operators is considered a significant source of risk. During normal activity, loss of skin scales by shedding is about $10^4\,\text{min}^{-1}$;

a large proportion of these skin scales will be contaminated with species of the normal skin flora [5]. A key point, however, is skin flora are mainly nonpathogenic micrococci, diphtheroids, and staphylococci. Other organisms (e.g., *Salmonella* and *Escherichia coli*), not part of the resident skin flora, may also be carried transiently on the skin surface and become a source of contamination [5]. This source of contamination is well recognized and manufacturers utilize good hygienic practices to control this source of bioburden.

Given these factors and contamination from skin flora is mainly nonpathogenic, the probability of viable pathogenic organisms is conservatively estimated at 0.5. P4 = 0.5 (5×10^{-1}).

Thus, the estimated overall probability of infection for the conservative case and more aggressive case of the examples above is shown in Table 7.9 for a terminal sterilization process of a process that can achieve an SAL of 10^{-6}.

The analysis alone (see also below) concludes in the conservative case scenario, there is a minor reduction in the overall probability of risk of infection while the more aggressive case predicts a substantial decrease in the risk of infection.

As noted in the introduction of Section 7.4.1, the application of this analysis could be applied for the special case of using an SAL of 10^{-4} for a product that cannot withstand sterilization to 10^{-6}. This is shown in Table 7.9B. The more aggressive case estimates an SAL of 10^{-6}. This puts into perspective the low patient risk of this scenario.

Table 7.9 An estimated overall probability of infection.

	Conservative case	**More aggressive case**
Panel (A)		
P1	1×10^{-6}	1×10^{-6}
P2	1	0.1 (1×10^{-1})
P3	1	0.2 (2×10^{-1})
P4	0.5 (5×10^{-1})	0.5 (5×10^{-1})
Overall probability	5×10^{-7}	1×10^{-8}
Panel (B)		
P1	1×10^{-4}	1×10^{-4}
P2	1	0.1 (1×10^{-1})
P3	1	0.2 (2×10^{-1})
P4	0.5 (5×10^{-1})	0.5 (5×10^{-1})
Overall probability	5×10^{-5}	1×10^{-6}

7.4.2 Other factors influencing the assurance of sterility

Other factors influencing the SAL or PNSU* should also be considered. These include:

7.4.2.1 Patient's immuno-compromised status and ability to treat the infection

The patient's condition may vary significantly. Elderly patients or patients with multiple comorbidities are more likely to exhibit a more compromised status and a decreased ability to fight off an infection. Some patients are given a prophylactic dose of antibiotics prior to treatment with the health-care product which improves their ability to resist infection. Many microorganisms are resistant to the medications that have traditionally been used to treat the infections caused by the organism. Multi-drug resistant organisms (MDRO) may be present impacting the ability of patients to be treated. It has been estimated up to 50% of antibiotics are ineffective in treating MDROs. The ability to treat patients is also influenced by the patient's failure to take antibiotics as prescribed.

7.4.2.2 Bioburden control in the manufacturing environment

As per nonquantifiable aspects of standards, manufacturers have implemented numerous controls for bioburden to help ensure adequate sterilization. These controls include:

- Environmental Monitoring to support controlled manufacturing environments. Typical monitoring includes viable air testing and viable surface testing. It should be noted that the level of controls for aseptic processing is significantly higher than that required for terminal sterilization.
- Utility systems are routinely monitored to ensure control of contamination in the controlled manufacturing environment. The manufacture of aseptically processed finished goods often takes place in controlled environments such as isolators.
- Typical engineering controls in these areas include the following. It should be noted again that the level of controls for aseptic processing is significantly higher than that required for terminal sterilization.
    - high-efficiency particulate air (HEPA) filtering of the incoming air,
    - differential pressure to direct airflow from the manufacturing area out to the ancillary spaces and beyond,
    - temperature and humidity control to ensure manufacturing area is not conducive to microorganism growth and for the comfort of the manufacturing operators,

- annual certification of classified spaces to ensure engineering controls are acceptable,
- routine maintenance of the heating, ventilation, and air conditioning (HVAC) system,
- facility housekeeping procedures typically include cleaning and refuse removal, frequency of cleaning, approved cleaning agents/chemicals, and documentation of these activities,
- pest control to prevent facility contamination by pests, and
- gowning procedures, which typically describe personal hygiene and gowning requirements, instructions for cleaning individual stations, associated equipment, and items being transferred into the controlled environment.

7.4.2.3 Sterilization validation methodology

Some sterilization validation methodologies provide extra assurance the PNSU★ requirement is met, as seen in the statistical analysis of the quantifiable aspects of a terminal sterilization overkill method (Section 7.3.5). There are other considerations that can be significant contributing factors to the assessment of patient risk, for example, when sterilizing a product at a PNSU★ of 10^{-4} because it cannot withstand a PNSU★ of 10^{-6}. These considerations add to confidence that such a terminal sterilization process will not result in significant risk to the patient.

An example of such a consideration is the conservative nature of the delivered dose compared to the sterilization dose in radiation sterilization. Terminal radiation sterilization processes result in a distribution of doses, not a homogeneous sterilization dose. Therefore product receives a range of doses as well as a range of SAL values. For instance, when applying a 20 kGy 10^{-6} sterilization dose, a dose range of 20–35 kGy is common and would likely provide a PNSU★ range of 10^{-6}–10^{-9} or less. This is illustrated in Fig. 7.14, the distribution of doses received in a radiation sterilization dose mapping validation. The maximum PNSU★ at the lowest dose received by the product (in this case just above 20 kGy taking uncertainty into account), is $<10^{-6}$. The SAL at the center of the dose distribution to the product, in this case approximately 28 kGy, is approximately 10^{-8}.

As noted in the introduction of Section 7.4.1, the application of this analysis could be applied for the special case of using an SAL of 10^{-4} for a product that cannot withstand sterilization to 10^{-6} as per Fig. 7.14B. This puts into perspective the low patient risk of this scenario; the SAL at the center of the dose distribution to the product, in this case approximately 21 kGy, is $<10^{-6}$.

7.4.3 Comparison to real-world infection rates

This clause puts the statistically quantifiable portion of patient risk from terminal sterilization, as discussed above, into the perspective of real-world health-care infection rates. As seen in Chapter 6, *Review of Current Practice in Preventing Health-care-Associated Infections*, neither packaging, aseptic processing nor terminal sterilization is significant contributors to real-world infection rates. Basic hygiene; standard procedural precautions; good practice with long-term access products, for example, urinary tract catheters, ventilators, and central lines; and reprocessing of complex devices in overworked central sterilization service departments are the focus of infection control.

A comparison of the potential for infection based on sterilization of health-care products, even at a PNSU* of 10^{-4}, to real-world infection rates reveals that medical devices are not the prevalent source of infection. As described in Chapter 6, a variety of sources contribute to the infection rates experienced by the patient, and thus rates may vary by hospital, region, and the type of devices used for treatment. As reported in Chapter 6, average HAIs are 4.5% in the US and 7.1% in the European Union. Rates in developing countries may be up to 30% and up to 66% in underdeveloped countries. It is estimated that half of HAIs are related to long-term use devices, for example, catheter-associated urinary tract infections (CAUTI).

Fig. 7.15 shows a comparison of hospital infection rates by source compared to the expected medical device infection rate based on the assumptions above. The data demonstrate the probability of patient infection due to device sterilization is orders of magnitude lower than those real-world rates experienced by the patient. A related analysis of the Center for Disease

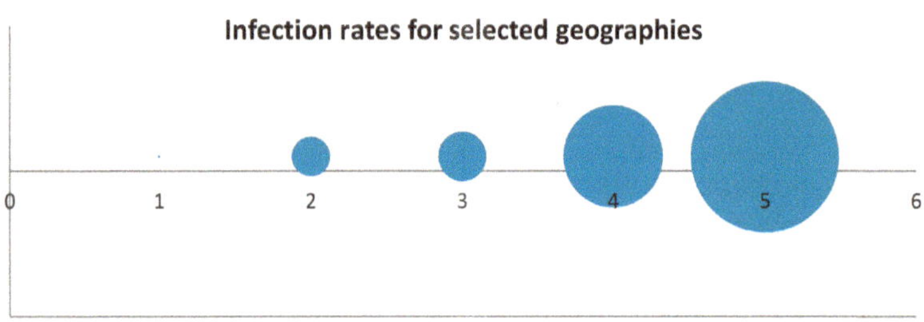

Fig. 7.15 Hospital infection rates vs medical device. Key: (1) Medical Device sterilized at PNSU* of 10^{-4}; (2) Estimated US HAI rate attributable to medical device[1]; (3) Estimated EU HAI rate attributable to medical device[1]; (4) Estimated HAI rate in developing countries due to medical device[1]; (5) Estimated HAI rate in underdeveloped countries due to medical device[1]. Note 1: literature rate divided by half to reflect the estimated long-term use device rate.

Control (CDC) surgical site infection relates in comparison with conservative infection rates from sterilized medical devices has been published [7].

7.5 Risk acceptability—Bringing it all together, the real risk to the patients

Stakeholders, that is, physicians, patients, and regulators, understand that the use of health-care products entails some degree of risk. The acceptability of a risk to a stakeholder is influenced by the likelihood of occurrence and the severity of the outcomes and by the stakeholder's perception of the risk. The decision to use a medical device requires the residual risks to be balanced against the anticipated benefits of the procedure. Such judgments should consider the intended use, performance, and risks associated with the medical device, as well as the risks and benefits associated with the clinical procedure or the circumstances of use.

Risk acceptability is determined by the manufacturer. Methods of determining acceptable risk include, but are not limited to, the following:

(a) Using applicable standards that specify requirements which, if implemented, will indicate achievement of acceptability for the applicable device relative to particular risks. This is the case with packaging, aseptic processing, and terminal sterilization as per the standards analyzed above. In the case of terminal sterilization, a PNSU* of 10^{-6} is deemed an acceptable risk (ISO 14971, EN 556-1 and AAMI ST67) based on the use of a recognized sterilization standard (see, for example, Table 7.4).

(b) Comparing levels of risk evident from medical devices already in use. Devices processed aseptically with UCBs as per Section 7.3.3 are deemed acceptable when terminal sterilization cannot be achieved.

(c) Utilization of clinical study data, especially for new technology or new intended uses, to demonstrate new benefits outweighs risks.

(d) Considering the state of the art and available information such as technology and practice existing at the time of design. "State of the art" is used here to mean what is currently and generally accepted as good practice.

Methods (b), (c), and (d) require an analysis of risk vs benefits. Acceptability is achieved with a favorable risk-benefit analysis.

Stakeholders may weigh risks and benefits using the following factors:

(a) Uncertainty

Uncertainty in the estimates of benefits and risks can be weighed. Consideration of the estimates for the occurrence of harms and the potential benefits of a new technology or device can be considered.

(b) Patient Impact
Risk to the patient may be increased if the device treatment or technology is not available.

(c) Product availability
Availability of a product or technology should be considered. Patients may benefit from new treatment modalities and technologies not currently available due to limitations based on sterilization methods. Patients and caregivers may prefer access to the device or technology.

(d) Types of benefits
The value that patients place on the benefits of new devices and technologies should be considered. New devices may address unmet needs.

(e) Magnitude of benefits
Consideration of the magnitude of the benefits should be considered. For example, the use of alternate PNSU★s could lead to more innovative products being available to patients.

(f) Probability of the patient experiencing one or more benefits
Different patient populations may experience more or fewer benefits. Benefits may vary across patient subgroups. New technologies may benefit subgroups with unmet needs.

(g) Duration of benefits
Duration of the benefit may vary. Consideration of the benefit achieved vs the risk should be considered.

(h) Consideration of the potential harms, for example, infection, sepsis, or even death should be considered. Are other complications possible? How likely is the infection to be treated?

(i) Patient factors
Consideration for the patient's willingness to accept the probable risks of the device or technology in exchange for the probable risks should be weighed. Use of Patient Preference Information, PPI, when available should be used. Consideration for the patient's understanding of the risks and benefits should be weighed.

(j) Alternative treatments
Consideration for other therapies and their availability to the patient and their effectiveness should be considered.

(k) Benefits to health-care professionals (HCPs) and caregivers
Access to new technologies or improved designs can improve device ease of use, and thus lower the potential for use errors. This is significant considering the increase in device usage by patients and caregivers.

7.6 Conclusion

This chapter places the quantification of patient risk in perspective across several industry sectors and in perspective relative to real-world infection rates in health-care facilities. Terminal sterilization is the preferred approach to minimizing the risk of infection due to bioburden on health-care products and has served the industry well for decades. Terminally sterilized product is packaged before sterilization and, if the packaging is developed and validated as per ISO 11607-1 and 11607-2, sterility is assured for the lifetime of the product As per ISO 13408-1, if terminal sterilization cannot be applied due to deleterious effects on product, aseptic processing may be applied. Aseptic processing has also served the industry well for decades. As per ISO TS 19930:2017, if terminal sterilization cannot be applied due to deleterious effects on product, another option can be utilized in addition to aseptic processing, a risk-based use of alternative SALs (PNSU*s in this chapter).

The use of a terminal sterilization SAL (PNSU*) of 10^{-6} has historically been deemed necessary, in general, because when attempting to set suitable microbial limits or standards for medical devices, the industry is faced with multiple and varied factors impacting safety, and cannot define precisely what level and types of product bioburden represent a hazard and what is safe [5]. A view across industry sectors, however, and a risk-based approach provides a new opportunity to manage risk effectively while creating new opportunities for new products and technologies.

The use of packaging standards to ensure robust processes to maintain sterility, and the use of sterilization standards to achieve terminal sterilization or validated aseptic manufacture of sterile product, has been demonstrated by history to achieve appropriate controls and consistently sterile product as intended. This is despite using quantifiable processes and sample sizes which do not always statistically achieve the intended PNSU*. However, a rigid implementation of the terminal sterilization expectation of a 1 in a million PNSU* has unintended consequences. The need to achieve a PNSU* of 10^{-6} can limit the development and introduction of new sensitive combination products, pharmaceutical, or biologic products. The result may be a reduced benefit to the patient and the inability to address unmet clinical needs. The use of higher PNSU*s, for example, 10^{-4}, however, can maintain acceptable risk and provide access to new technologies with minimal impact to the patient based on the potential of infection from a contaminated device. Data and analysis of this chapter demonstrate the added risk is extremely unlikely while the potential for new and innovative treatment options is significant. It seems warranted, therefore, to support the likelihood of innovative new health-care products reaching patients with sterility assurance innovation. An example of this innovation is the clarification of the risk-based use of alternative SALs (lower PNSU*s in this chapter) while maintaining acceptable risk to the patient is discussed in Chapter 9.

References

[1] M.S. Favero, Patient infections:The relevance of sterility assurance levels, in: Sterilization of Medical Products,Vol.VI, 3, Polyscience Publications, Morin Heights (Canada), 1993, pp. 156–163.
[2] M.S. Favero, Sterility assurance: concepts for patient safety, in: W.A. Rutala (Ed.), Disinfection, Sterilization and Antisepsis: Principles and Practices in Healthcare Facilities, Association for Professionals in Infection Control and Epidemiology, Washington, DC, 2001, pp. 110–119. chapter 12.
[3] Bryans TD, Kimbrell M, Darnell R, Hitchins VM, Lappalainen S, Liu D, and Masefield J. Sterility Assurance Levels for Terminal Sterilization of New/Emerging Healthcare Products, CDC Conference, 2010, Poster # 1841.
[4] An example of a legacy paradigm from steam sterilization is addressed in a series of articles by J.P. Agalloco, Increasing patient safety by closing the sterile production gap, Parts 1–3, PDA J Pharm Sci Tech 71 (2017) 261–278.
[5] S.P. Denyer, R.M. Baird (Eds.), Guide to Microbiological Control in Pharmaceuticals and Medical Devices, second ed., 2007.
[6] E. Scott, S.F. Bloomfield,The survival and transfer of microbial contamination via cloths, hands and utensils, J. Appl. Bacteriol. 68 (1990) 271–278.
[7] S.W. Srun, B.J. Nissen, T.D. Bryans, M. Bonjean, Medical device SALs and surgical site infections: A mathematical model, Biomedical Instrumentation & Technology (2012). May/June 2012.

CHAPTER 8

Developing new products

Stan Lam
Process and Technology Development, Stryker Neurovascular, Fremont, CA, United States

Contents

8.1 Background

The development of single use combination devices is driven by user needs. Research and development teams identify opportunities such as controlled drug delivery, biodegradability, or electronic data acquisition to improve patient outcomes, treat new conditions, or increase patient compliance. For implantable devices, sterility is assumed and is the minimum barrier to entry. This hurdle is cleared while attempting to address patients' unmet needs. This will typically be captured in the design control process when defining the user needs requirements. During the development cycle, the development team generates a general sterilization strategy and constantly assesses if the product functionality is adversely impacted by the sterilization process. As the product design evolves, generating more data demonstrating that product performance is maintained after sterilization, confidence that the product is compatible with the sterilization modality will also increase. As the product takes form, challenge sterilization conditions should also be assessed.

Assurance of Sterility for Sensitive Combination Products and Materials
https://doi.org/10.1016/B978-0-12-805082-8.00008-6

The development of a sterilization process impacts both product safety and cost. It is essential to develop a robust sterilization process that ensures a continuous supply of the product in the market.

Validation of sterilization methods using established methods [1], such as dry heat, moist heat, ethylene oxide, and radiation sterilization, has been extensively applied in the medical device industry and is covered in detail in Chapter 3 of this book. This chapter focuses on the thought process for developing the sterilization strategy for challenging sensitive combination products. The assessment of the viability of a product concept should be done early. The amount spent during the development of a product can easily run into seven figures per quarter. Failing late has a major impact on large companies and may jeopardize smaller organizations.

8.2 Sterilize at 10^{-6} SAL

The sterilization strategy should be prioritized early in the program. This enables the product design to be modified or the sterilization modality be changed early on while minimizing the impact on the overall timelines. The avoidable wasted time, people, and capital resource would be indefensible if the project is terminated with a fully functioning device that cannot be sterilized. The strategy allows the team to identify additional resource and time requirements to develop a robust sterilization process.

Products that are similar to existing products or line extensions are relatively straightforward to leverage the existing sterilization methodology. With the experience of the organization, the process can be developed quickly and efficiently. The overall risk is low because of the experience in developing sterilization processes for the product as well as the ability to leverage the existing infrastructure around quality, supply chain, and operations.

Products that are new to the organization but similar to other products in the marketplace have a medium overall risk. Although the technical risk is low, the execution risk is high. Substantial work is required to identify suppliers, establish the quality infrastructure, develop and document procedures and processes, train employees, and work out the logistics required to implement a new sterilization modality.

The highest risk products are both novel and have little or no precedent within the organization. This class of products has high resource and timeline risk. De-risking the program as soon as possible increases the probability of success and allows timeline risk to be accurately estimated. Technical risk is prioritized as the complexity and novelty of the product increases uncertainty. An early literature review to evaluate material compatibility with the various sterilization modalities will avoid the more costly build and test strategy. This may provide an efficient and quick assessment as to whether a 10^{-6} SAL is achievable.

The Association for the Advancement of Medical Instrumentation (AAMI) has published an excellent resource "Compatibility of materials subject to sterilization" TIR17:2017 [2], which enables the developer to prioritize sterilization modalities based on general material compatibility guidance. Initial testing of clinically relevant performance outputs will help confirm risks and identify if additional resourcing would be required to develop the product. Evidence that the product cannot be sterilized to a level of 10^{-6} SAL must be provided before other strategies such as aseptic processing or an alternative SAL can be used.

Even after proof of principle has been confirmed, the development of a robust and efficient sterilization process is important for the successful development of the product. Ideally, if a pre- and poststerile correlation of functional performance can be established, then the sterilization process can proceed in parallel to the nonsterile device development. Often, however, the relationship cannot be established because of the high variability in the output. If the impact of sterilization on the output cannot be quantified, then all the developmental studies that relate to those outputs will require sterilization. Since the preliminary sterilization process is typically not optimized for efficiency, increased delays directly impact the critical path of the program.

As the data package is being collected, other criteria such as the stability of the product under accelerated aging at the sterilization process challenge limits should be gathered to understand the robustness of the product to the sterilization conditions. Accelerated aging is important because it is a long lead time item. Challenge limits such as maximum acceptable dose for radiation sterilization and challenge sterilization cycles for ethylene oxide sterilization further aids in the assessment of the sterilization risk.

In all three cases, terminal sterilization to 10^{-6} SAL is the default, unless it can be demonstrated that it is unachievable. Only after it can be demonstrated that terminal sterilization at 10^{-6} SAL cannot be achieved can an alternative SAL or aseptic processing can be utilized. The aseptic process and the alternative terminal sterilization SAL process have taken slightly different approaches to the demonstration that a product cannot be sterilized.

The difference in approach reflects the evolution as aseptic processing was often associated with pharmaceuticals and the alternative SAL approach was developed for medical devices. Aseptic processing has demonstrated a long history of delivering safe products to the patient, while alternative SAL has inherent benefits in the statistical rigor. This is covered extensively in Chapter 7.

8.3 Aseptic processing

The first biologic, a recombinant insulin Humilin developed, approved, and sold by Genentech/Lilly in the United States in 1982 [3], is still on the market today. ISO 13408-1:2008 [4] was developed to help provide guidance for these aseptic processed products. A similar approach was used by the European Medicines Agency (EMA) [5]. The demonstration that a 10^{-6} SAL is unattainable is a prerequisite for aseptic processing. One strategy is to follow the EMA approach [5] to document this. The product is systematically assessed as summarized in Figs. 8.1 and 8.2, which have been reproduced from the EMA guidelines [5]. For some materials, such as biologics, that are known to be incompatible with terminal sterilization, a literature review may suffice. For other products, the strategy will depend on whether the product is aqueous or nonaqueous based.

For aqueous-based products, steam sterilization should be explored. If this sterilization modality is not successful, alternative methods for bioburden reduction such as sterile filtration and terminal microbial reduction processes should be used whenever possible in conjunction with aseptic manufacturing (Fig. 8.1).

Nonaqueous-based products should explore different terminal sterilization modalities. The flowchart in Fig. 8.2 does not explicitly identify EO as a modality because the EMA guidance document [5] assumes that most powders will not be compatible. Assessment of other sterilization modalities such as lower radiation doses using Method 1, Method 2, or Method VD_{max} should be completed. If these methods are demonstrated not to be successful, sterile filtration and other bioburden reduction processes should be considered in conjunction with aseptic manufacturing.

With this information in hand, an assessment can be made to identify both the risks and benefits for an aseptic processed product knowing that the due diligence was first performed to have a terminally sterilized product.

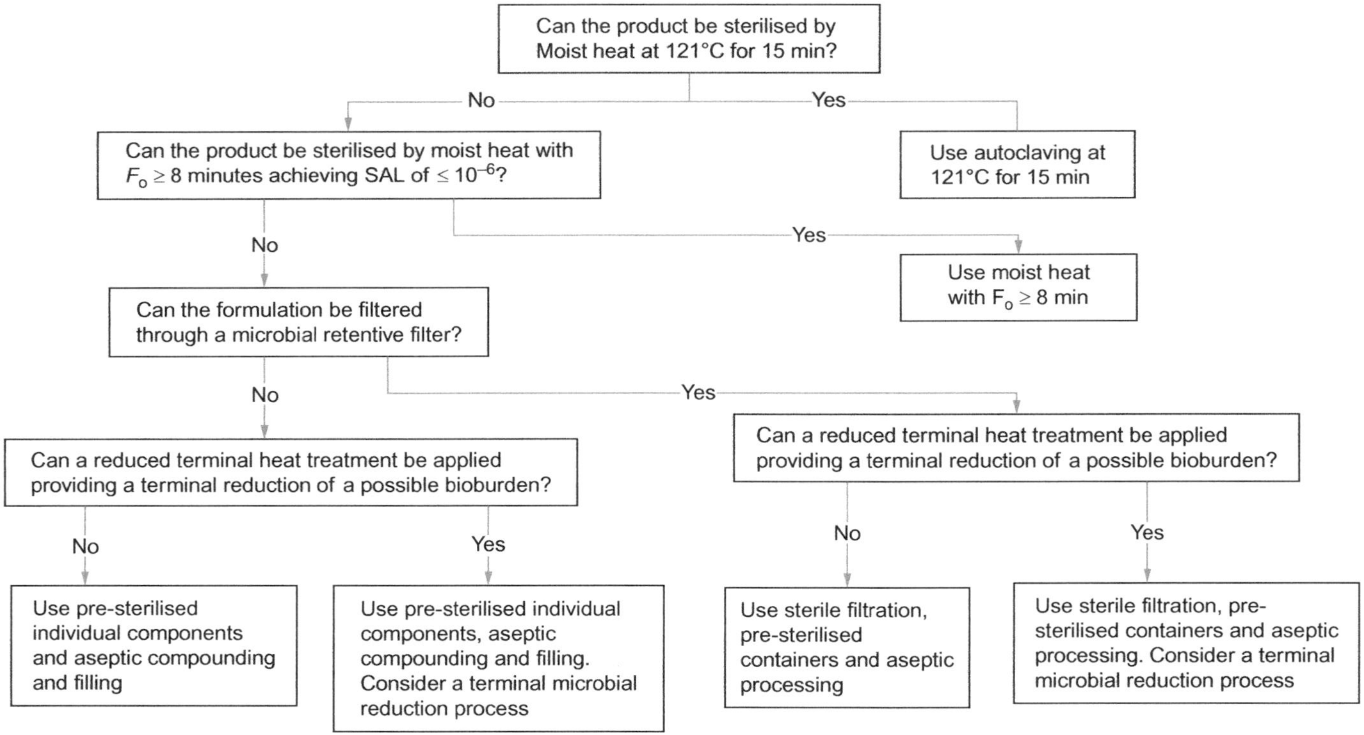

Fig. 8.1 Decision tree for sterilization choices for aqueous products. *From EMA/CHMP/CVMP/QWP/850374/2015 Guideline on the sterilization of the medicinal product, active substance, excipient and primary container, April 2016, European Medicines Agency.*

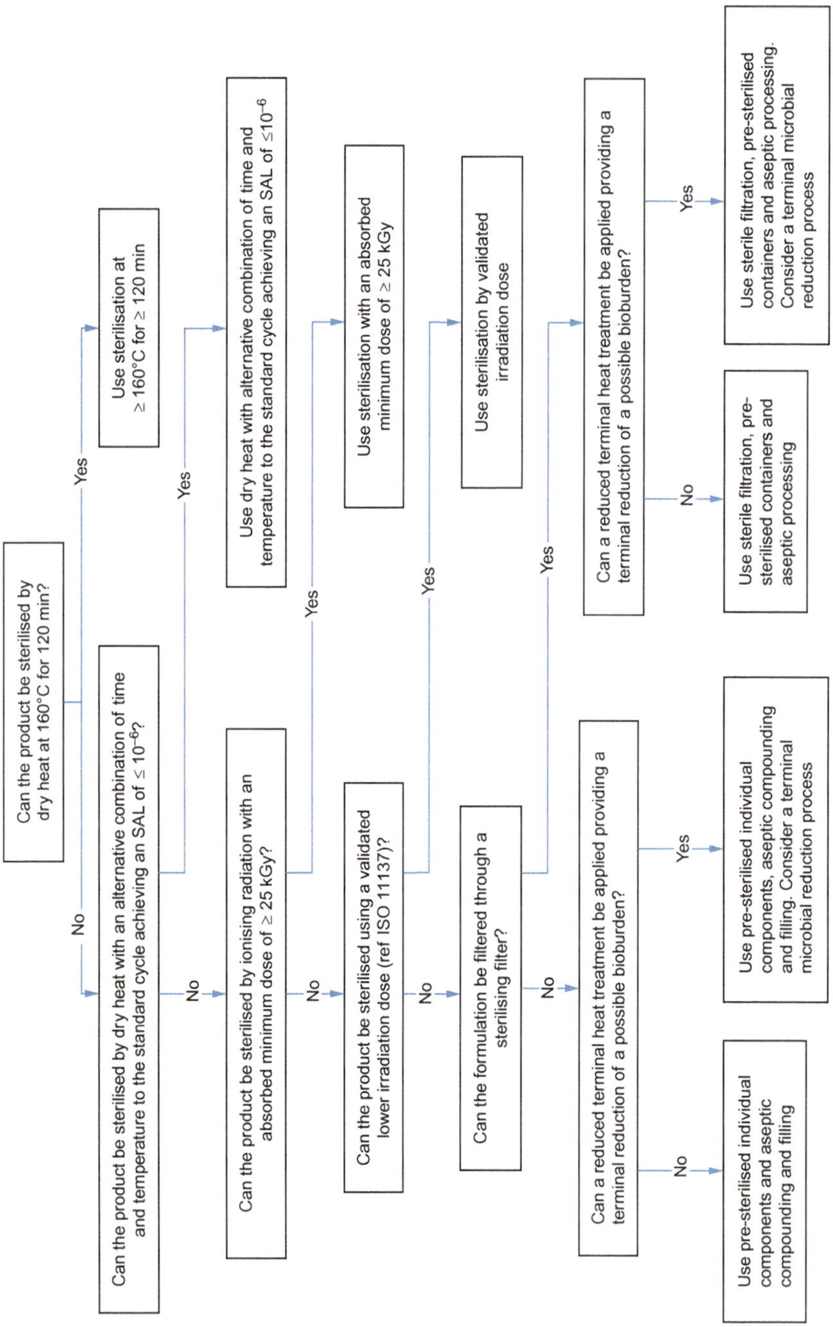

Fig. 8.2 Decision tree for sterilization choices for nonaqueous liquid, semisolid, or dry powder products. *From EMA/CHMP/CVMP/QWP/850374/2015 Guideline on the sterilization of the medicinal product, active substance, excipient and primary container, April 2016, European Medicines Agency.*

8.4 Alternative SAL

The alternate SAL approach is governed by ISO/TS 19930:2017 [6], and the recently updated document provides more specificity on the evidence required to justify using a higher SAL. The alternative SAL approach has been residing predominantly in the medical device arena and is outlined in Fig. 8.3. Understanding the material compatibility with the various sterilization modalities is the first step.

ISO/TS 19930 provides a framework to systematically attempt to achieve a terminal sterilization at 10^{-6} SAL. These strategies can be grouped into improving device compatibility with the sterilant, reducing the exposure time that the sterilant is in contact with the device, and reducing bioburden, which in turn reduce exposure to reach a 10^{-6} SAL. Higher SALs are considered only after demonstrating that these strategies were ineffective.

8.4.1 Improving device compatibility

Sterilants inactivate bioburden indiscriminately by reacting with any available functional groups. This reactivity is not limited to the bioburden but also any susceptible groups on the components of the device itself. The component functionality after sterilization depends on the component-sterilant interaction, the criticality of the component, and the stresses and strains imparted to the component. Alternative component materials should be considered if the sterilization cycle compromises the function of the component. Changing materials is significantly easier if the design changes occur earlier in the program before significant data is generated.

Another strategy to improve device compatibility would be to use an alternative sterilization modality. Changing materials may not an option if a given component is critical to the design. An alternative sterilization modality may be necessary. This topic has been addressed by the FDA in "Submission and Review of Sterility Information in Premarket Notification [510(k)] Submissions for Devices Labeled as Sterile: Guidance for Industry and Food and Drug Administration Staff" [1]. The first step would be an assessment of Established Category A methods. Category A methods—heat (dry and moist), ethylene oxide, and radiation (e-beam or gamma)—have a long history of use in the medical device industries with published consensus standards. Depending on previous experience with the sterilization modality and the device, this assessment can range from literature searches to design of experiments to map the design space.

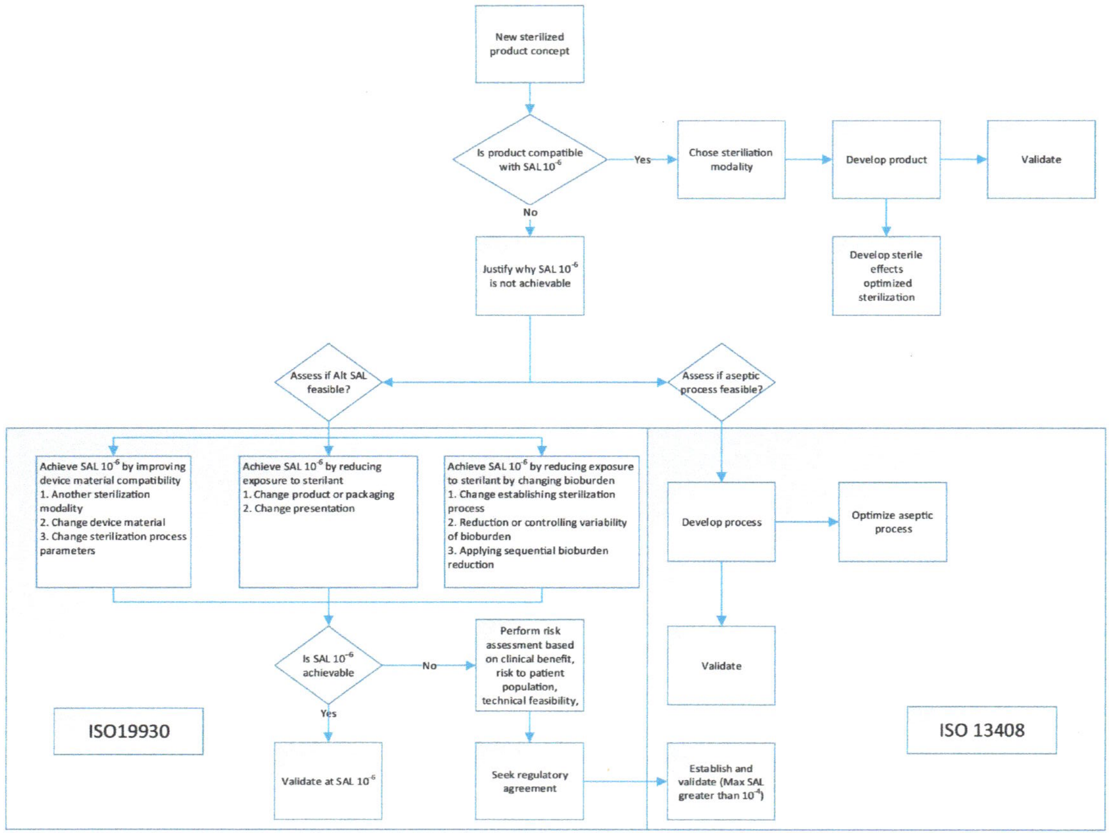

Fig. 8.3 Flowchart outlining approaches for alternative SAL or aseptic processing.

A third alternative approach to minimize the impact of sterilization on the component is to alter the sterilization conditions. Reduction of temperature or exposure time may be effective solutions for most sterilization modalities. For example, if temperature during exposure is an issue, moving from gamma radiation to e-beam can enable the product to be realized. The documented justification why alternative established sterilization modalities are not viable options is an integral part of the due diligence to justify alternate SALs.

8.4.2 Reducing exposure time

The second approach to achieving a 10^{-6} SAL is to explore packaging changes or sterile load configurations that will reduce the exposure time. Understanding how the product and packaging interacts with the sterilizer provides the sterilization professional critical process parameters or leavers to impact component compatibility. For example, product is exposed to a distribution of doses during radiation sterilization. Understanding the dosing at a granular level enables the sterilization professional to modify the load configuration to narrow the distribution of dose (maximum to minimum). This allows a reduction in both the nominal as well as the maximum dose. For ethylene oxide sterilization, the duration of the cycle is dependent on the diffusion of the sterilant into the product. Changing the design of the packaging to increase the area of Tyvek to increase the gas exchange or decreasing the path length of narrow channels can reduce overall exposure times of the product to the sterilant.

8.4.3 Reducing bioburden

The third option, reducing the bioburden load, enables an alternative approach to reducing exposure time. Bioburden-based sterilization validation methods achieve a 10^{-6} SAL based on the initial bioburden. Reduction in the average bioburden enables lower exposure to achieve a given SAL. The distribution of bioburden is typically non-normal with just a few units having orders of magnitude higher levels of microbes than the rest of the population of units. A single unit with a high bioburden load can have a disproportionately large impact on the averages. Minimizing these "high fliers" can significantly reduce the sterilizing dose.

A key to improved bioburden control is to understand their sources. Microbial monitoring is invaluable to develop effective controls. Common sources of contamination control include raw material controls, gowning and handling procedures, and presterilization of subassemblies. An alternate method to establish the sterilization process is another approach particularly if the natural bioburden is more susceptible to the sterilant than a biological indicator. The guidance documents for all sterilization processes (ISO 11135, ISO 11137, ISO 17665, or ISO 20857) have bioburden-based methodologies, but the additional characterization of the natural bioburden population is more resource intensive and costly.

Finally, an alternative option is to sequentially reduce bioburden. This is especially effective if the bioburden is due to incoming material that is outside of the immediate control and the sensitive components are added later in the process. This strategy involves identifying the major sources of bioburden, isolating those components, and presterilizing. Overall bioburden is reduced if the appropriate controls are implemented during the final product assembly.

8.4.4 Other SAL options

Alternative SAL strategy development requires the documentation of the systematic assessment outlined in Sections 8.4.1–8.4.3 to demonstrate a 10^{-6} SAL was explored and not technically feasible. This assessment, however, is only half of the equation. The benefits of the device to the patient also needs to be identified. A meaningful discussion with regulatory bodies can only occur after both the risks and the benefits are understood.

8.4.4.1 Identifying the risks

The 10^{-6} sterility assurance limit is the gold standard. For some difficult to sterilize products, this may not be achievable. A systematic approached, such as strategies outlined in Section 7 of ISO/TS 19930:2017, should be used to demonstrate a 10^{-6} SAL could not be achieved.

8.4.4.2 Identifying the benefits

An informed decision requires both the risks and the benefits to be understood. The product definition along with how it meets unmet patient needs must be assessed. What is the purpose of the product and what is the competitive landscape? What is the indication for use and what is the implication if not treated? Does this improve patient outcome or compliance, and what is the impact of noncompliance? These key questions enable the risk to be taken in context.

8.5 Conclusion

The development of sterile single use medical products, both devices and pharmaceuticals, can have a significant impact on the patient's quality of life. Scientists and engineers from both industry and regulatory bodies have worked together to ensure that the treatments offered to patients are safe and effective. Both terminal sterilized as well as aseptic processed single use medical products have a long history of patient safety. The theoretical benefits of a sterile product processed to a 10^{-6} SAL over an aseptic process product are clear: minimizing the risk to the patient. From a practical perspective, however, aseptic processed products, with the appropriate controls in place, are extremely effective and safe. Although these innovative products provide new treatment options to patients, it is becoming increasingly challenging to sterilize them to the same SAL. ISO/TS 19930-1:2017 and ISO 13408-1:2008 provide a framework where due diligence to ensure risk is minimized is balanced with the challenges of the difficulties in sterilizing the new sensitive combination products.

References

[1] FDA, Submission and Review of Sterility Information in Premarket Notification [510(k)]. Submissions for Devices Labeled as Sterile Guidance for Industry and Food and Drug Administration Staff, 2016, https://www.fda.gov/downloads/ucm109897.pdf.

[2] AAMI TIR17, Compatibility of Materials Subject to Sterilization, 2017.

[3] C. Quianzon, I. Cheikh, History of insulin, J. Community Hosp. Intern. Med. Perspect. 2 (2) (2012) https://doi.org/10.3402/jchimp.v2i2.18701.

[4] ISO 13408-1, Aseptic Processing of Health Care Products—Part 1: General Requirements, 2008.

[5] European Medicines Agency, EMA/CHMP/CVMP/QWP/BWP/850374/2015 Draft: Guideline on the Sterilization of the Medicinal Product, Active Substance, Excipient and Primary Container Aseptic Processing, 2016.

[6] ISO/TS 19930:2017 Guidance on aspects of a risk-based approach to assuring sterility of terminally sterilized, single-use health care product that is unable to withstand processing to achieve maximally a sterility assurance level of 10^{-6}.

CHAPTER 9

Regulatory pathway for labeling combination products as sterile☆

Trabue D. Bryans[a], Eamonn Victor Hoxey[b], Steven Turtil[c]
[a]BryKor, LLC, Marietta, GA, United States
[b]E V Hoxey Ltd, Cirencester, United Kingdom
[c]U.S. Food and Drug Administration/CDRH, Silver Spring, MD, United States

Contents

☆The sections of this chapter entitled "Seeking FDA feedback" and "FDA guidance on labeling devices as sterile" have been authored by Steven Turtil. They reflect the views of the author and should not be construed to represent FDA's views or policies.

Assurance of Sterility for Sensitive Combination Products and Materials
https://doi.org/10.1016/B978-0-12-805082-8.00009-8

9.1 Labeling products as sterile

One of the most challenging hurdles for combination products or products sensitive to standard sterilization processes is understanding the requirements for making a claim in the labeling of the product that it is sterile and the regulatory pathway to making such a claim. The broad assumption in the industry is that if a combination or sensitive product cannot be sterilized to a maximal sterility assurance level (SAL) of 10^{-6} using traditional sterilization processes, it automatically must be manufactured using aseptic processing. Several standards, such as International Standards Organization (ISO) 13408-1 and European Agency for the Evaluation of Medicinal Products (EMA) guidance of the sterilization of medicinal products, state that terminal sterilization is preferred for providing sterile product, with aseptic processing being an option if terminal sterilization is not possible. To that end, new guidelines are available that facilitate the understanding of and provide guidance in situations when terminal sterilization at an SAL other than 10^{-6} might be acceptable.

There are several standards and guidance documents that provide options for achieving a sterile label claim, including Pharmacopeias, European Standards (EN) and EMA documents, United States (US) standards and US Food and Drug Administration (FDA) ISO guidance documents. The EN documents that are utilized in many countries around the world are EN 556-1 and EN 556-2. The central US document is AAMI ST67. In addition, in the ISO arena, ISO TS 19930 provides guidance for meeting the requirements of EN 556 and AAMI ST67, whereas the ISO 13408 series provides comprehensive guidance for achieving a sterile claim using aseptic processing. A current list of FDA-recognized, consensus standards is available at https://www.accessdata.fda.gov/scripts/cdrh/cfdocs/cfStandards/search.cfm.

9.1.1 Communicating with regulatory authorities

Regardless of the choice of a sterile label claim or the means by which it is achieved, regulatory bodies for specific countries have the authority to approve the processes chosen for supporting that claim. Therefore, it is critical to understand the regulatory pathway that pertains to a particular country or region for supporting and obtaining approval for a label claim that the product is sterile.

Each country's regulatory authority has a system for submitting a product for approval. Integral to that approval is the sterile label claim and mechanism by which it is supported. Information is provided on the submission pathway for regulatory authorities in the European Union (EU) and the United States.

9.2 Seeking FDA feedback

In 2019, the FDA published the guidance document "Requests for Feedback and Meetings for Medical Device Submissions: The Q-Submission Program—Guidance for Industry and Food and Drug Administration Staff." This guidance is intended to provide a summary of the pathways available to industry for early collaboration and discussions about medical device submissions with the Center for Devices and Radiological Health (CDRH) and the Center for Biologics Evaluation and Research (CBER). It is available at: https://www.fda.gov/downloads/medicaldevices/deviceregulationandguidance/guidancedocuments/ucm311176.pdf.

This guidance document presents the methods through which industry can request feedback from or a meeting with the FDA via Q-Submissions or Q-Subs. Q-Subs can be related to various types of premarket submissions such as:

- Investigational Device Exemption (IDE) applications,
- Premarket Approval (PMA) applications,
- Humanitarian Device Exemption (HDE) applications,
- Premarket Notification [510(k)] Submissions,
- Clinical Laboratory Improvement Amendments (CLIA) Waiver by Applications (CW),
- Dual 510(k) and CLIA Waiver by Application Submissions (Duals),
- Accessory Classification Requests, and
- certain Investigational New Drug Applications (INDs) and Biologics License Applications (BLAs).

Q-Subs are requests for interaction with FDA regarding potential or planned medical device submissions, potential or planned device-led combination product submissions, as well as issues communicated in marketing submission hold letters, Investigational Device Evaluation (IDE) letters, Clinical Laboratory Improvement Amendments (CLIA) Waiver by Applications (CW) hold letters, and certain Investigational New Drug (IND) Clinical Hold letters.

There are several different types of Q-Subs that provide mechanisms to request FDA interaction and which are discussed in this guidance document. Some of these include Pre-Submissions, Informational Meetings, Study Risk Determinations, and Submission Issue Requests.

The Q-Submission Program provides the opportunity for interaction with the FDA from the early stages of device design through the regulatory process, while supporting the FDA's goal of facilitating new medical device development. The guidance presents an overview of the various types of Q-Subs available through the FDA, as well as general timeframes, methods of feedback, and additional information.

One type of Q-Sub, known as a Pre-Submission (Pre-Sub) is a request for FDA feedback prior to an intended premarket submission (i.e., IDE, PMA, HDE, De Novo request, 510(k), Dual, BLA, IND), Accessory Classification Request, or CW. Pre-Subs include specific questions for which feedback is provided in the form of a written response or a written response followed by a meeting in which any additional feedback or clarifications are documented in meeting minutes. These meetings may take the form of teleconferences or in-person meetings.

The Agency will, after reviewing the information, develop feedback to address the submitted questions and, if a meeting is requested, work with the submitter to determine a mutually agreeable meeting date and time.

9.2.1 Additional points to consider

For several reasons, it is highly encouraged that industry begin communicating early with the FDA, and with the right component of the Agency. For some particular types of devices the Agency may have issued a device-specific guidance with recommendations that differ from those of other device types. Similarly, there may be FDA-recognized standards that have special sections or annexes dedicated to a particular device type (e.g., ethylene oxide residual limits for intraocular lenses).

Upon initially contacting the Agency, it might be determined that developing a benefit-risk analysis in support of any departure from established standardized practices could be of great value. Such an approach could be applied to proposed alternatives to standardized sterility assurance levels, the use of alternative sterilants and sterilization methods, or inclusion of alternative and unique device materials. Such an analysis should address the principle factors that would likely be taken into consideration during the premarket review process—including an evaluation of risks (and risk mitigation measures) and anticipated benefits associated with the proposed approach. Consulting FDA guidance documents that address the factors to consider when making benefit-risk determinations for PMAs and De Novo classifications, and for IDEs, could be useful.

The FDA guidance documents do not establish legally enforceable responsibilities, but rather describe the Agency's current thinking and practices and should be viewed only as recommendations.

9.3 EU submission process

9.3.1 Regulatory classification

There is not a specific category of combination products in EU regulations; products are categorized as either medicinal products or medical devices depending on their principle mode of action. Products that combine a medicinal product or substance and a medical device are regulated under the Medical Devices Directive (Directive 93/42/EEC), the Medical Devices Regulation (Regulation EU 2017/745), or the Directive for medicinal products (Directive 2001/83/EC). Essentially, if the principle mode of action is physical, for example, a drug-coated stent, this would be classified as a device but if the principle mode of action is pharmacological or immunological, for example, a syringe pre-filled with a biopharmaceutical for administration, it would be classified as a medicinal product. The legislative acts for devices and medicinal products are intended to ensure appropriate interaction involving combination products in consultations during premarket assessment and of exchange of information from postmarket oversight.

It is important to be aware that the Medical Devices Directive, which was implemented in 1993, is in transition to be replaced by the Medical Devices Regulation. The Medical Devices Regulation came into force in May 2017 with a 3-year transition period until application in May 2020. In particular, the Medical Devices Regulation amends the Directive on medicinal products in relation to applications for marketing authorization of medicinal products that integrate a medical device element.

Any device that is intended to administer a medicinal product is governed by the Medical Devices Regulation unless it takes the form of a single integral product. Such an integrated product would be intended to administer a medicinal product exclusively in the given combination and would not be reusable. Such an integral product is governed by the Directive on medicinal products or Regulation (EC) No 726/2004, which established the EMA, as applicable. When an integral device is covered by a marketing authorization for a medicinal product, the relevant general safety and performance requirements set out in the Medical Devices Regulation apply as far as the safety and performance of the device part of the single integral product are concerned. Furthermore, the application for a marketing authorization has to include either:

- a manufacturer's declaration of conformity or relevant certificate from a notified body designated under the Medical Devices Regulation allowing the manufacturer to CE-mark the device, supplied on its own, under this regulation; or,
- an opinion on the conformity if the device part with the relevant general safety and performance requirements of the Medical Devices Regulation, provided by a notified body designated under the Medical Devices Regulation.

Any device that incorporates as an integral part a substance with an action ancillary to that of the device which, if used separately, would be considered to be a medicinal product, including a medicinal product derived from human blood or human plasma, is assessed and authorized in accordance with the Medical Devices Regulation. Such a product would be categorized as a Class III device and require review by a notified body designated under the regulation. As part of the process of review to obtain that certificate, this notified body would consult with a competent authority for medicinal products in one of the EU member states in regards to the safety, quality, and usefulness of any substance considered to be a medicinal product.

Other changes brought in by the Medical Devices Regulation affect gaps in coverage of the Advanced Therapy Medical Products Regulation [Regulation (EC) No 1394/2007] and Directive 2004/23/EC regarding human tissues and cells. Any product containing human material was excluded from the Medical Devices Directive. Products manufactured utilizing derivatives of tissues or cells of human origin that are nonviable or are rendered nonviable now come under the scope of the Medical Devices Regulation if they meet the definition of a medical device.

9.3.2 Marketing authorization as a medical product

Applications for market authorization as a medicinal product could be made by a centralized procedure through the EMA or a decentralized procedure through national competent authorities, depending on the nature of the medical product and the market strategy of the applicant for market authorization. The procedures and methods applied to assure sterility of the product would be detailed in the portion of the submission generally referred to as the Chemistry, Manufacturing, and Controls (CMC) section.

The review of the submission would consider the sterility requirements in relation to the applicable monographs of the European Pharmacopeia. Any submission that did not follow the European Pharmacopeia's expectation of terminal sterilization achieving a maximal sterility assurance level of 10^{-6} would be subject to individual review.

Competent authorities for medicinal products and the EMA offer pre-submission meetings where the rationale for decisions made in regard to assurance of sterility could be discussed.

9.3.3 CE-marking for a medical device

The regulatory system for medical devices offers a variety of routes for conformity assessment based on the risk classification of the medical device and the strategy for regulatory compliance developed by the manufacturer.

All devices, irrespective of their risk classification, have to meet the general requirements for safety and performance that apply to them. In terms of sterile devices, the applicable requirements are that the device:

(a) is designed, manufactured, and packed in a nonreusable pack and/or according to appropriate procedures to ensure that it is sterile when placed on the market and remains sterile, under the storage and transport conditions laid down, until the protective packaging is damaged or opened;

(b) is manufactured in appropriately controlled environmental conditions;

(c) is manufactured and sterilized by an appropriate, validated method;

(d) is labeled with the word 'STERILE' or an accepted symbol indicating sterility;

(e) has packaging and/or labeling that distinguishes between identical or similar product sold in both a sterile and a non-sterile condition.

The regulatory requirements for devices indicate that devices, systems, or processes that are in conformity with relevant harmonized standards are presumed to be in conformity with those requirements of the regulations covered by those standards. References to standards that are considered to be harmonized are published in the Official Journal of the European Union. The list of harmonized standards under the Medical Devices Directive includes standards identifying requirements for terminally sterilized medical devices to be designated sterile, EN 556-1, and the European adoptions of international standards for the development, validation, and routine control of sterilization by the methods of sterilization generally applied for terminal sterilization. It is expected that these same standards will be given the status of harmonized under the Medical Devices Regulation.

Any device incorporating a medicinal product would be classified as a Class III medical device under the classification rules (Rule 14 of Annex VII of the Medical Devices Regulation). The manufacturer has to prepare and sign a declaration of conformity in order to CE-mark the device. In order to sign such a declaration for a Class III device, the manufacturer would require certification from a notified body of review of a design dossier or type test. Both these approaches require the notified body to review the manufacturer's technical documentation. The requirements for the technical documentation are set out in Annex II of the Medical Devices Regulation. Aspects of the technical documentation relevant to claims or sterility are as follows:

- Design and manufacturing information
  - **(a)** information on design and development stages applied to the device;
  - **(b)** information and specifications on the manufacturing processes and their validation;
  - **(c)** identification of all sites, including suppliers and subcontractors, where design and manufacturing activities are performed.
- General safety and performance requirements

Information for the demonstration of conformity with the general safety and performance requirements that are applicable to the device taking into account its intended purpose together with justification, validation, and verification of the solutions adopted to meet those requirements.

The demonstration of conformity includes:

(a) the general safety and performance requirements that apply to the device and an explanation as to why others do not apply;

(b) the method or methods used to demonstrate conformity with each applicable general safety and performance requirement;

(c) the harmonized standards or other solutions applied; and.

(d) the documents providing evidence of conformity with the harmonized standard or other method applied to demonstrate conformity with the general safety and performance requirements.

Notified bodies offer pre-submission meetings where the rationale for decisions made in regards to assurance of sterility could be discussed.

9.4 FDA guidance on labeling devices as sterile

The FDA has published guidance specifically for information to be provided in 510(k) submissions for devices labeled as "sterile." This document was published in 2016, and is entitled "*Submission and Review of Sterility*

Information in Premarket Notification (510(k)) Submissions for Devices Labeled as Sterile" ("510(k) sterile devices guidance"). This guidance is intended to provide a summary of the information that the Agency recommends applicants include in 510(k) submissions to CDRH and CBER for devices intended to be labeled as sterile. The guidance is available at: https://www.fda.gov/downloads/medicaldevices/deviceregulationandguidance/guidancedocuments/ucm109897.pdf.

The 2016, 510(k) sterile devices guidance updates and clarifies the information in its 2002 predecessor, "*Updated 510(k) Sterility Review Guidance K90-1*" and it provides expanded guidance related to recent advances in sterilization technology. Until established to be otherwise, such sterilization technology innovations are considered to have the potential of increasing human health risks. One of these is the risk of infection, if a new technology does not provide adequate sterility assurance. This guidance provides clarification regarding the Agency's concerns and expectations.

It is worth noting at the onset that the scope of this guidance includes medical devices that are intended to be labeled sterile as a result of being subjected to "*industrial terminal sterilization processes based on microbial inactivation*" rather than microbial exclusion. Accordingly, methods such as filtration and aseptic processing are outside of the scope of this guidance.

Should an applicant wish to impart a specific sterility assurance to a device using a unique sterilization method as part of an innovative approach to processing a sensitive device, the following summary of the 2016, 510(k) sterile devices guidance is provided to help identify concerns associated with the development of unique sterilants, unique combinations of sterilants, and/or unique sterilization methods. (For other submission types such as PMAs and IDEs for devices that raise similar issues, industry should ~~to~~ reach out to the Agency to obtain case-by-case, relevant guidance.)

9.4.1 Methods of sterilization

One area of clarification provided by this guidance is the refined definitions of the three categories of industrial sterilization methods. The basis of these definitions is multifactorial, and the category designation of any given technology has the potential to change as the Agency's knowledge of the process increases with experience.

- Established A methods are those for which there is a well-established and extensive history of safe and effective use, and extensive literature, including the existence of dedicated, FDA-recognized, consensus standard(s).

- Established B methods are those for which there is a history of safe and effective use, albeit a relatively shorter one, and for which there are no dedicated, FDA-recognized, consensus standards. In short, the Agency has confidence in the safety and effectiveness of a specific process with clearly defined, discrete parameters, and not necessarily all permutations of that method.
- Novel methods are those for which there is inadequate information to conclude that the process is effective to support a sterile label claim, or to assure that processed devices are safe and effective for its intended use. The evaluation of the validation data will likely help the Agency ascertain the effectiveness of the proposed process.

9.4.2 Content recommendations for 510(k)s

The information that should be included within a 510(k) submission has evolved from that specified in the earlier versions of this guidance (1990 and 2002), but the basic areas of documentation have not changed. Two significant areas of expansion are evident in the 2016 guidance; the guidance now recommends that sufficient information be provided to ensure that the Agency can identify the sterilization method category, and to ensure that bacterial endotoxin pyrogenicity concerns are adequately addressed.

The information of interest to the Agency at the time of submission covers five areas. It is recommended that submissions include:

1. A description of the sterilization method. Guidance is significantly expanded in this section, recommending submission of a more specific description of the sterilization method to help the Agency ascertain the method category. Additionally, the inclusion of information on the radiation dose if that method is to be used, or sterilant residuals information if a chemical sterilant is to be used, is recommended.
2. A description of the method used to validate the proposed cycle, as well as citations for all relevant and/or dedicated FDA-recognized consensus standards. The Agency recommends that applicants use FDA-recognized consensus standards for all general process validation testing, where available. A current list of these standards is available at https://www.accessdata.fda.gov/scripts/cdrh/cfdocs/cfStandards/search.cfm.
3. The SAL specification. While a majority of medical devices are imparted with a maximal SAL of 10^{-6}, a maximal SAL of 10^{-3} may be sufficient for some devices that are intended to contact only intact skin. The guidance specifically states: "*For questions related to alternative SALs, we recommend direct consultation and pre-submission meetings with FDA*"

and directs the reader to FDA's, "*Requests for Feedback on Medical Device Submissions: The Pre-Submission Program and Meetings with Food and Drug Administration Staff*" guidance document (previously cited).

4. A description of the pyrogenicity testing, if applicable. Guidance is significantly expanded in this section, which identifies the general categories of devices for which pyrogenicity testing should be performed, and cites relevant references to guidance and standards. In addition, it recommends that the submission should include information on the test method and acceptance criteria. Finally, it recommends that the submission should include more extensive information on alternatives to batch testing, if that route is intended.
5. A description of the sterile barrier system(s). This should be provided, as well as a simple description of any simulation methods (e.g., distribution, accelerated aging) and test methods (e.g., dye penetration, seal strength) used to validate package integrity and shelf life claims.

9.5 Documents pertaining to terminal sterilization and SAL

9.5.1 Guidance from the Association for the Advancement of Medical Instrumentation

The Association for the Advancement of Medical Instrumentation (AAMI) has had a standard in place since 2006, which has been recognized by FDA and which addresses SALs other than 10^{-6}. The current edition is titled AAMI ST67: 2019: *Sterilization of health care products—Requirements and guidance for selecting a sterility assurance level (SAL) for products labeled "sterile."* However, a revision is in process, most likely due to be published in 2019.

AAMI ST67 allows for SALs other than 10^{-6}, such as 10^{-5}, 10^{-4}, and 10^{-3}, depending on whether the product can tolerate traditional sterilization processes. Historically, alternative SALs have been more accepted in the United States because the North American medical device industry and the CDRH of the FDA have applied two SALs to describe assurance of product sterility—an SAL of 10^{-6} for products intended to contact breached or compromised tissue, and 10^{-3} for products not intended to come into contact with breached skin or compromised tissue.

As in ISO TS 19930, everything presented in AAMI ST67 is based on the premise that a manufacturer will pursue sterilization to a maximal SAL of 10^{-6} before considering other options. However, AAMI ST67 provides more in-depth guidance into what a manufacturer should consider when evaluating whether sterilization to a 10^{-6} SAL is feasible/reasonably practicable for a particular product. Points to consider as far as feasibility include extent of research or development, length of time for regulatory approval, effect of modifications, extent of supporting studies or testing, supply chain availability, and other points associated with practicality of an extensive delay or redesign.

The revision of AAMI ST67 that is in process will include several changes and additions to the current version. One main change is that ST67 will more closely harmonize with ISO TS 19930 in language, format, and inclusions. AAMI ST67 not only embraces the guidance in ISO TS 19930 but also provides, as a national standard, requirements that can be used to support the choice of an alternative SAL.

As in ISO TS 19930, the ultimate goal in AAMI ST67 is to seek an appropriate balance between the clinical benefit of a product and patient safety and the scale of risk and feasibility of what might be required in resources versus logistics to sterilize to a maximal SAL of 10^{-6}, compared to using an alternative SAL or selecting aseptic processing.

Regarding AAMI ST67, ISO 13408, and any future published standards, the FDA maintains a searchable database of current "FDA-recognized consensus standards" at https://www.accessdata.fda.gov/scripts/cdrh/cfdocs/cfStandards/search.cfm. This database enables the user to determine if a standard is currently FDA-recognized, and if so, it provides the user with a "Supplemental Information Sheet" (SIS). The SIS will enable the user to identify the edition of the standard that is recognized based on publication date, identify the individual subparts that are recognized (e.g., part 1, 2, or 3), and provide additional valuable information in the "Extent of Recognition" and "Relevant FDA Guidance and/or Supportive Publications" sections.

9.5.2 European standards for terminal sterilization

EN 556-1, Sterilization of medical devices—Requirements for medical devices to be designated "STERILE"—Part 1: Requirements for terminally sterilized medical devices was initially published in 1994 to provide requirements for designating devices as sterile that would be consistent across all methods of terminal sterilization. EN 556-1 was updated in 2001 without changing the core requirement, a corrigendum was issued in 2006 and the standard was subsequently reconfirmed without change. EN 556-1 has been harmonized under the Medical Devices Directive and is expected to be harmonized under the Medical Devices Regulation. EN 556-1 has been adopted by countries outside of the EU, including ~~by~~ Australia, China, Israel, and South Africa.

EN 556-1 has a single requirement, that for a terminally sterilized medical device to be designated "STERILE", the probability of there being a viable microorganism present on/in the device is equal to or less than 1×10^{-6}. Compliance with this requirement is the demonstrated provision of documentation and records which demonstrate that the devices have been subjected to a validated sterilization process fulfilling this requirement.

While complying with a harmonized standard such as EN 556-1 provides a presumption of conformity with applicable regulatory requirements, following a harmonized standard is not mandatory. A note in EN 556-1 indicates that permission for acceptance of a probability greater than that specified can be sought through the appropriate regulatory bodies. The note continues by indicating that such permission depends on the individual situation, including consideration of the risk management activities undertaken by the manufacturer of the medical device. The corrigendum to the standard that was issued in 2006 was to update the cross reference in the note to EN ISO 14971, the standard for risk management for medical devices. EN 556-1 does not provide any additional guidance on situations where a greater sterility assurance level might be accepted or the detailed considerations that would need to be addressed in such circumstances. ISO TS 19930 was prepared with the intention of providing such guidance and experts from several European countries participated in its preparation.

In contrast to AAMI ST 67, EN 556-1 does not indicate that there is acceptance of application of a maximal sterility assurance level of 10^{-3} for certain devices based on their intended use not coming into contact with breached skin or compromised tissue.

9.5.3 New guidance from ISO

The most recent guidance concerning assurance of sterility and SAL is ISO TS 19930: 2017, *Guidance on aspects of a risk-based approach to assuring sterility of terminally sterilized, single-use health-care product including that unable to withstand processing to achieve maximally a sterility assurance level of 10^{-6}*. This guidance was developed to provide information that could be used to meet ~~the~~ Note ~~in~~ 4.1 of EN 556-1: 2001, which specifies that permission for acceptance of a sterility assurance level of greater than 10^{-6} (e.g., 10^{-5}) may be sought through appropriate regulatory bodies, with risk management by the manufacturer being required. ISO TS 19930 also provides information in this regard to meet the requirements in "clauses" 4.2.4 of AAMI ST67: 2019.

The scope of ISO TS 19930 is clear in that it does not specify an SAL to be used in circumstances where a product cannot be sterilized to a 10^{-6} SAL.

The choice of an alternative SAL and the support of that choice depend on risk assessment and the applicable regulatory authority. The document does, however, provide much guidance associated with options for achieving a maximal SAL of 10^{-6}. Some of the options presented in the document that might be pursued in determining whether a product can be sterilized to a maximal SAL of 10^{-6} include assessment of product design, materials, validation approaches, sterilization methods, and bioburden reduction. One or more of these options might allow a sterilization process that can achieve a maximal SAL of 10^{-6}.

A significant inclusion in the document is a flow chart that guides the user through the process of determining whether a product can be sterilized to a maximal SAL of 10^{-6} and, if not, what should be done to support the selection of an alternative SAL. Risk management is a main theme in supporting the choice of an alternative SAL and guidance is given for areas to be addressed, including risk management considerations and risk management output. In addition, ISO TS 19930 contains a section on Label Claims that discusses the regulatory requirements that apply for a product to be labeled sterile and again emphasizes that labeling a product as sterile is typically subject to national or regional regulations or standards.

The ISO TS 19930 guidance points out that clinical benefit must be weighed against other technical and logistical factors in order to determine whether a product can or should be sterilized to a maximal SAL other than 10^{-6} SAL.

9.5.4 Documents pertaining to aseptic processing and assurance of sterility

The introduction of ISO 13408-1, as well as the decision tree provided in the EMA guidance on sterilization of medicinal products, clearly indicate that terminal sterilization is the preferred method of providing assurance of sterility, and, if terminal sterilization cannot be achieved, aseptic processing should be used. Terminal sterilization is preferred because it applies a process that inactivates microorganisms rather than using procedures that prevent the introduction of microorganisms. Consequently, an active process that ensures a maximal sterility assurance level of 10^{-5}, 10^{-4}, or 10^{-3} could be considered as an option to using aseptic processing.

9.5.5 ISO 13408 series

The ISO 13408 series of standards specifically addresses aseptic processing and the many requirements associated with that approach to provide a sterile product. Although aseptic processing is typically associated with pharmaceutical and biological products, ISO 13408-7 addresses aseptic manufacturing of combination products, products that might use both terminal sterilization and aseptic processing, or similar products that are typically manufactured in small batches. The validation in these cases is limited to performing process simulations that incorporate the largest batch size manufactured. Hence it must be recognized that the assurance of sterility provided by validation using these lesser batch numbers will not be the same as that provided by traditional 1000 or 10,000 unit runs of the typical pharmaceutical manufacturer.

9.5.6 EN 556-2

EN 556-2, Sterilization of medical devices—Requirements for medical devices to be designated "STERILE"—Part 2: Requirements for aseptically processed medical devices was published in 2003. This standard parallels EN 556-1 in respect of sterile medical devices that are prepared by aseptic processing. This standard was revised in 2015 to update the references to the European adoption of the ISO 13408 series of standards for aseptic processing.

EN 556-2 requires control of a number of factors in order designate aseptically processed medical devices as sterile. These factors relate to controls and/or records of:

- the manufacturing environment
- the sterilization of components
- the competence of personnel
- interventions in the process
- the performance of process simulations
- inspections and tests of finished product

The acceptance limits and actions for occurrence of non-sterile units in process simulations in initial performance qualification and periodic requalification are the same as those in ISO 13408-1.

Compliance with EN 556-2 is shown by providing documentation and records of the validation and routine control of the aseptic process.

9.5.7 Evaluation of medicinal products

The draft revision of the EMA decision trees for the selection of sterilization methods, Guideline on the sterilization of the medicinal product, active substance, excipient, and primary container (EMA/CHMP/CVMP/QWP/BWP/850374/201), indicates that terminal sterilization is preferred to aseptic processing. This draft guidance states that terminal sterilization provides the highest assurance of sterility and should be used whenever possible. It continues by stating that for highly sensitive products such as biological products where terminal sterilization of the product is not possible, aseptic processing under controlled conditions provides a satisfactory quality of the medicinal product and that the use of aseptic processing can be accepted in certain situations even if the formulation itself can be terminally sterilized if other benefits are gained for the patients or users of the product.

9.6 Summary

There are standards and guidelines associated with providing sterile healthcare products that could provide optimal pathways for sterility assurance of innovative new products for patients worldwide. It is the task of the manufacturer to investigate the options and possibilities before selecting a course of action. Integral to that approval is the sterile label claim and mechanism by which it is supported, because the final authority for approving a claim of sterile resides with the regulatory authority of a particular country or region. For manufacturers and regulators alike, the ultimate goal is patient safety, therefore selecting the means of delivering sterile product requires knowing the options, assessing the risks associated with each option, complying with applicable regulations, and then determining the approach that creates the best outcome for the patient, the product, and the company.

Further reading

[1] Directive 2001/83/EC of the European Parliament and of the Council of 6 November 2001 on the Community Code Relating to Medicinal Products for Human Use (OJ L 311, 28.11.2001, p. 67).
[2] Directive 93/42/EEC of 14 June 1993 Concerning Medical Devices (OJ L 169, 12.7.1993, p. 1).
[3] Regulation (EU) 2017/745 of the European Parliament and of the Council of 5 April 2017 on Medical Devices, Amending Directive 2001/83/EC, Regulation (EC) no 178/2002 and Regulation (EC) no 1223/2009 and Repealing Council Directives 90/385/EEC and 93/42/EEC (OJ L 117, 5.5.2017, p. 1).
[4] Regulation (EC) No 1394/2007 of the European Parliament and of the Council of 13 November 2007 on Advanced Therapy Medicinal Products and Amending Directive 2001/83/EC and Regulation (EC) no 726/2004 (OJ L 324, 10.12.2007, p. 121).
[5] Directive 2004/23/EC of the European Parliament and of the Council of 31 March 2004 on Setting Standards of Quality and Safety for the Donation, Procurement, Testing, Processing, Preservation, Storage and Distribution of Human Tissues and Cells (OJ L 102, 7.4.2004, p. 48).

[6] Regulation (EC) No 726/2004 of the European Parliament and of the Council of 31 March 2004 Laying down Community Procedures for the Authorisation and Supervision of Medicinal Products for Human and Veterinary Use and Establishing a European Medicines Agency (OJ L 136, 30.4.2004, p. 1).

[7] European Medicines Agency, EMA/CHMP/CVMP/QWP/BWP/850374/2015, Guidance on the sterilization of the medicinal product, active substance, excipient and primary container.

[8] ISO TS 19930: 2017 Guidance on aspects of a risk-based approach to assuring sterility of terminally sterilized, Single-Use Health Care Product Including that Unable to Withstand Processing to Achieve Maximally a Sterility Assurance Level of 10^{-6}.

[9] AAMI ST67: 2019, Sterilization of Health Care Products – Requirements and Guidance for Selecting a Sterility Assurance Level (SAL) for Products Labeled "Sterile".

[10] ISO 13408-1: 2006, Aseptic processing of health care products—Part 1: General requirements.

[11] ISO 13408-7: 2012, Aseptic processing of health care products—Part 7: Alternative processes for medical devices and combination products.

[12] EN 556-1:2001, Sterilization of Medical Devices — Requirements for Medical Devices to Be Designated "STERILE"—Part 1: Requirements for Terminally Sterilized Medical Devices.

[13] EN 556-2:2015, Sterilization of Medical Devices—Requirements for Medical Devices to Be Designated "STERILE"—Part 2: Requirements for Aseptically Processed Medical Devices.

[14] FDA Guidance Document, "Factors to Consider When Making Benefit-Risk Determinations for Medical Device Investigational Device Exemptions", 2017.

[15] FDA Guidance Document, "Factors to Consider When Making Benefit-Risk Determinations in Medical Device Premarket Approval and De Novo Classifications", 2016.

[16] FDA Guidance Document, "Requests for Feedback and Meetings for Medical Device Submissions: The Q-Submission Program—Guidance for Industry and Food and Drug Administration Staff", 2019.

[17] FDA Guidance Document, "Submission and Review of Sterility Information in Premarket Notification (510(k)) Submissions for Devices Labeled as Sterile – Guidance for Industry and Food and Drug Administration Staff", 2016.

CHAPTER 10

Path forward

Byron J. Lambert[a], Joyce M. Hansen[b]
[a]Assurance of Sterility Task Force, ASTF, Abbott, Temecula, CA, United States
[b]J&J Sterility Assurance, Johnson & Johnson, Raritan, NJ, United States

Contents

10.1 What is next with combination products?

Chapter 2 highlighted that combination products and biologics for regenerative medicine are bringing increased value to patients and increased need for creative sterility assurance solutions. In broader context, combination products, pharmaceuticals, and biologics are key for finding innovative solutions to the most challenging and pervasive unmet clinical patient needs in neuroscience, oncology, cardiology, and pulmonary disease. These four areas alone represent untold human suffering and a &45T economic burden to society [1].

Combination product opportunities for meeting patient needs and related challenges for assuring sterility are further elevated with bioabsorbables, microelectronics, and multiple active agents. Sterility assurance professionals need to facilitate these innovative products with timely solutions for sterility assurance challenges so that the pipeline of new products for needy patients is not unnecessarily restricted.

https://doi.org/10.1016/B978-0-12-805082-8.00010-4

10.2 Sterility assurance landscape in the 2020s

Sterility assurance has many challenges; ongoing and new solutions are required for

- high volume sterile commodity products that keep health-care facilities meeting the needs of patients worldwide;
- now common combination products such as Drug Eluting Stents (DES) and prefilled syringes;
- innovative and complex combination products with development time scales of 5–15 years that do not have simple sterility assurance solutions; and
- all forms of personalized regenerative biologics and cell therapy products that may require transformative approaches to sterility assurance.

This picture is complicated by current and future realities of the terminal sterilization technology landscape. Moist heat, radiation, and ethylene oxide sterilization have been the workhorses of the industry for decades, with the latter two dominating the market for heat-sensitive health-care products. Both radiation and ethylene oxide technologies are experiencing market pressure; 80% of the radiation sterilization market uses gamma radiation sterilization utilizing the isotope cobalt 60. There continues to be manufacturing, transportation, disposal, and terror threats related to this technology. Electron beam and x-ray radiation sterilization are alternative technologies but often include cost concerns, especially with commodity products [2]. Ethylene oxide sterilization is increasingly under pressure from environmental health and safety perspectives [3]. Although alternative gas technologies are available, they are still in the early stages of the development to meet supply chain needs.

Innovation and new sterility assurance paradigms are required on many fronts. Required sterility assurance focus areas include new sterility assurance technologies (Chapters 3 and 4), a pan-industry risk framework (Section 10.3), and highly competent sterility assurance professionals (Section 10.4).

10.3 Pan-industry sterility assurance risk framework

To meet the needs of patients for innovative new products, sterility assurance professionals need to see beyond the boundaries of their industry segment. The first step toward this broader patient-focused sterility assurance approach is seeing what the patient cares about: receiving valuable new products in a timely manner while reducing the risk of infection.

10.3.1 Sterility assurance risks in health-care facilities

To reduce the risk of infection around the world, the greatest need for patients is increased focus on and innovation in reducing health-care associated infections (HAI). As highlighted in Chapter 6, the realities of 2%–30% infection rates in health-care facilities is a staggering risk to patients and families and financial burden to health-care systems. Ongoing focus on basic controls related to hygiene, good hospital practices, and consistent long-term wound care continue to be critical. Discerning analysis and collaborative solutions are required.

Directly related to HAI is sterilization within the health-care facilities in central sterilization departments, and in particular, sterilization of reprocessed devices. Reusable devices such as endoscopes can be challenging to disassemble, clean, and sterilize with tragic results when operational pressures lead to poor practices (e.g., insufficiently trained sterility assurance staff succumbing to time pressures from overbooked operating theaters). There has been significant focus and progress related to device design and process standardization in this area [4], and ongoing diligence in this complex area is critical.

These compelling concerns need to get framed appropriately in order to pave the way for what could be a new wave of very valuable products for patients that could be manufactured directly in health-care facilities—regenerative medicinal biologic products. This opportunity also frames the need for innovation in the broader product development and regulatory paradigms being developed. There is a compelling need for clarity and thoughtfulness for sterility assurance professionals.

10.3.2 Sterility assurance risks related to single-use products

Moving out of the health-care facility, the sterility assurance professional needs to put the risks related to terminal sterilization and aseptic processing into broad perspective. When validated and controlled appropriately, terminal sterilization provides reproducible and validated logarithmic reduction of product microbial load while being contained in sterile barrier systems that prevent further contamination. This provides very high confidence in robust sterility assurance. It is the preferred approach to provide sterile product [5].

As discussed in Chapter 3, established moist heat, ethylene oxide, and radiation sterilization technologies have served the terminal sterilization industry well for decades. The industry has significant innovation within these established options as well as a growing array of technology options for terminal sterilization [6].

When terminal sterilization at a sterility assurance level of 10^{-6} is not possible, the well-traveled option that has also served the industry well for decades is aseptic processing (Chapter 4). When validated and controlled appropriately, aseptic processing maintains the sterility of sterile components and produces sterile finished goods within sterile barrier systems/container closure systems that do not allow further contamination. Innovation in this industry segment is providing technologies and environments in which it is increasingly simple and robust to combine sterile components into sterile products.

In addition to aseptic processing for product that cannot be terminally sterilized at an SAL of 10^{-6}, the less well-traveled option is the use of alternative SALs. As discussed in Chapter 9, this option was recently framed within ISO [7] and has been available longer through Association for the Advancement of Medical Instrumentation (AAMI). The increased clarity in this option of providing reliable and acceptable sterility assurance for needed products should well serve the industry as well as the patients. Chapter 7 enhances this clarity by providing a unique and broad perspective on how validation sample sizes for packaging, aseptic processing, and terminal sterilization fit into, but are not the whole story, for assuring sterility.

10.4 What is next for sterility assurance professionals?

The final area of sterility assurance focus to support innovation in meeting patient needs is highly competent sterility assurance professionals. Within health-care facilities, professionals experience enormous challenges under the pressure of immediate care for patients. This requires great competence and is likely the most important point of focus for patients from an infection risk mitigation perspective.

10.4.1 End-to-end sterility assurance

Sterility assurance professionals in industry providing single-use products are well served by a broad understanding of all industry segments. This can be understood in a framework of the entire product life cycle or 'end-to-end sterility assurance.' In the product R&D planning phase, knowing the innovation within established terminal sterilization technologies as well as innovation in novel sterilization technologies optimizes the opportunity to find a sterility assurance solution with a sterility assurance level of 10^{-6}. When this is not possible, knowing the innovation within aseptic processing and the clarified alternative SAL approach optimizes the chance of delivering valuable new products to meet patient needs.

Patients do not benefit from an R&D solution, however. They benefit when that solution is implemented to bring them an innovative sterile product. The sterility assurance professional needs to source the solution and then develop a robustly validated process. (S)he also needs to implement a robust supply chain with contingency since sterilization is a single point of supply chain failure. In addition, the SA (sterility assurance) professional needs to understand the process and the business deeply in order to appropriately address process and product exceptions that challenge the supply chain.

Coupled with all of this is the reality that all sterile products require robust sterile barrier systems to maintain sterility over time. Interfacing with the design of robust and sterilization compatible packaging for the shelf life of the product is critical (see Chapter 5).

10.4.2 Bringing it all together in a risk management framework

Bringing innovative product to market with robust sterility assurance will never be easy. The sterility assurance professional needs to pull all the above factors into a deep understanding of the product development process and risk management (see Chapter 8). As highlighted in Chapter 7, a simplistic approach will not be sufficient. All the inputs and risks need to be assessed in a risk-based framework that allows patient needs to be prioritized. This requires well-rounded, experienced, and collaborative sterility assurance professionals to seize the opportunities being provided for the patient. This is being made possible with increasing pan-industry forums provided in the industry. For example, Johnson and Johnson resurrected the Kilmer conference in 2016 to bring together thought leaders from the regulatory agencies, industry, and academia. In addition, they donated the proceedings of the Kilmer conference from 1974 to 2003 to AAMI to provide resources to the sterilization community [8].

10.5 What is next for the patient?

Confidence in a flow of valuable and innovative products facilitated by sterility assurance professionals minimizing the risk of infection is the key. Advances in biologics, personalized medicine, and new sensitive combination products will open new products and treatments to patients. A thorough understanding of the balance of risks to benefits and the options available to the sterility assurance professional is necessary. Nothing else will suffice!

References

[1] John Capek, IMRP 2016 presentation, referencing WHO, McKinsey 2012-02-27 ABT Newport Global Growth Presentation.
[2] J.W. Chou, M. Skornicki, J.T. Cohen, Unintended consequences of the potential phase-out of gamma irradiation, F1000 Research 7 (2018) 348.
[3] Guideline for Disinfection and Sterilization in Healthcare Facilities (2008) Center for Disease Control and Prevention. https://www.cdc.gov/infectioncontrol/guidelines/disinfection/sterilization/etheylene-oxide.html. Accessed: August 2, 2019.
[4] Food and Drug Administration (FDA), Reprocessing Medical Devices in Health Care Settings: Validation Methods and Labeling. Accessed: August 2, 2019.
[5] ANSI/AAMI/ISO 13408-1:2008 (R2017)/A1:2013 "Aseptic Processing of Health Care Products Package".
[6] Food and Drug Administration (FDA), January 21, 2016, Submission and Review of Sterility Information in Premarket Notification (510(k)) Submissions for Devices Labeled as Sterile: Guidance for Industry and Food and Drug Administration Staff.
[7] International Organization for Standards, ISO/TS 19930:2017 "Guidance on aspects of a risk-based approach to assuring sterility of terminally sterilized, single-use health care product that is unable to withstand processing to achieve maximally a sterility assurance level of 10^{-6}".
[8] Kilmer Conference Proceedings, http://www.aami.org/productspublications/content.aspx?ItemNumber=2594. Accessed August 2, 2019.

Index

Note: Page numbers followed by *f* indicate figures, *t* indicate tables, and *b* indicate boxes.

P

Q

R

S

Kolibri 360 GmbH
Ferdinand-Jühlke-Straße 7
99095 Erfurt, Deutschland
produktsicherheit@kolibri360.de